Transcatheter Aortic Valve Replacement

A. Claire Watkins • Anuj Gupta
Bartley P. Griffith

Transcatheter Aortic Valve Replacement

A How-to Guide for Cardiologists and Cardiac Surgeons

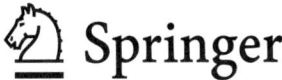 Springer

A. Claire Watkins
Department of Cardiothoracic
Surgery, Stanford University
School of Medicine
Stanford, CA
USA

Anuj Gupta
Division of Cardiology
University of Maryland, School
of Medicine
Baltimore, MD
USA

Bartley P. Griffith
Division of Cardiac Surgery
University of Maryland, School
of Medicine
Baltimore, MD
USA

ISBN 978-3-319-93395-5   ISBN 978-3-319-93396-2   (eBook)
https://doi.org/10.1007/978-3-319-93396-2

Library of Congress Control Number: 2018947376

Printed on acid-free paper

This Springer imprint is published by the registered company Springer
International Publishing AG part of Springer Nature.
The registered company address is: Gewerbestrasse 11, 6330 Cham, Switzerland

Contents

1 **Introduction** 1
   References 1

2 **Relevant Clinical Trials** 3
   References 8

3 **Valves Available in the United States** 13
   SAPIEN 3 13
   EVOLUT Pro 15
   References 18

4 **Preoperative Evaluation: Indications**
   and Risk Analysis 19
   Class I Recommendations 19
   Class IIa Recommendations 20
   Class IIb Recommendations 20
   Class III Recommendation: No Benefit 20
   Contraindications 23
   Bicuspid Aortic Valve 24
   Valve-in-Valve 25
   References 28

5 **Preoperative Imaging** 35
   Bicuspid Aortic Valve 40
   Valve-in-Valve 41
   References 42

6 Self-Expanding Versus Balloon-Expandable Devices 45
References 47

7 Valve Sizing 49
References 51

8 Aortic Access Planning and Procedures.......... 53
Transapical 53
Subclavian.................................... 56
Carotid 58
References 58

9 Wires, Catheters, and Cath Lab Rules 61

10 Procedural Considerations and Technical Details 69
Roles of Participants 69
Femoral Vessel Access......................... 69
Femoral Artery Closure Devices................ 71
Pacing 72
Pigtail Placement and Heparinization............ 73
Crossing the Aortic Valve...................... 74
Pre-TAVR Balloon Aortic Valvuloplasty 76
SAPIEN 3 Delivery System 77
Evolut Pro Delivery System.................... 79
Second Time-Out.............................. 80
SAPIEN 3 Deployment 81
Evolut Pro Deployment 85
Assessment and Management of Perivalvular Leak 88
References 90

11 Cardiopulmonary Bypass and Cardiac Surgery in TAVR............................. 91
Annular Rupture.............................. 93
Ventricular Injury 94
Aortic Injury.................................. 95

ECMO in TAVR 96
Steps for Emergent Femoral ECMO
Cannulation 98
Surgical TAVR Explantation 99
References 100

12 **Vascular Complications of TAVR** 103
References 107

13 **Medical Management and Complications
Following TAVR** 109
References 113

14 **Conscious Sedation for TAVR**................. 117
References 118

15 **Durability of TAVR**......................... 119
References 120

16 **Interesting and Complicated Cases**............. 121
Ventricular Perforation....................... 121
Coronary Occlusion.......................... 122
Annular Rupture 124
Moderate-Severe Paravalvular Leak............. 125
References 126

Index 129

Chapter 1
Introduction

As the most common valvular disease treated by cardiac surgeons, severe aortic stenosis (AS) carries a significant mortality, with a 50% risk of death over a 2-year period once patients develop significant breathlessness [1]. Since the first transcatheter aortic valve replacement (TAVR) performed in a non-operable patient in 2002 [2], both the study of its clinical use and the development of improved technologies have risen substantially. TAVR therapy is not only an option for 40% of patients considered high risk for surgical aortic valve replacement (SAVR) [3] but is also undergoing investigation for use in low-risk patients. As a cardiothoracic surgeon or interventional cardiologist, it is imperative that you master contemporary TAVR skills in order to offer total care of aortic valve disease. This manual provides the underlying fundamentals of TAVR, including basic information, procedural details, and surgical considerations, to enrich your learning as you scrub on your first or fiftieth TAVR.

References

1. Otto CM. Timing of aortic valve surgery. Heart. 2000;84:211–8.
2. Cribier A, Eltchaninoff H, Bash A, Borenstein N, Tron C, Bauer F, Derumeaux G, Anselme F, Laborde F, Leon MB. Percutaneous transcatheter implantation of an aortic valve prosthesis for

© Springer International Publishing AG, part of Springer Nature 2018
A. C. Watkins et al., *Transcatheter Aortic Valve Replacement*,
https://doi.org/10.1007/978-3-319-93396-2_1

calcific aortic stenosis: first human case description. Circulation. 2002 Dec 10;106(24):3006–8.
3. Iung B, Cachier A, Baron G, Messika-Zeitoun D, Delahaye F, Tornos P, Gohlke-Bärwolf C, Boersma E, Ravaud P, Vahanian A. Decision-making in elderly patients with severe aortic stenosis: why are so many denied surgery? Eur Heart J. 2005 Dec;26(24):2714–20.

Chapter 2
Relevant Clinical Trials

The PARTNER (Placement of Aortic Transcatheter Valves) trial is a series of trials that included the first prospective, randomized study to demonstrate the safety and non-inferiority of TAVR against medical therapy in inoperable patients and against SAVR in high-risk but operable patients. This consort diagram depicts the design of the study [1], including mortality results (Fig. 2.1):

The **PARTNER B** cohort consisted of 358 patients deemed inoperable by 2 surgeons experienced in high-risk SAVR who were randomized to TAVR or medical therapy. This study was done with the Edwards SAPIEN THV (a first-generation device). Although the Society of Thoracic Surgeons (STS) risk score was not an inclusion criterion for the trial, (the average score was 11.6%), many were inoperable secondary to comorbidities including porcelain aorta, chest radiation, severe COPD, or severe frailty. Both 1- and 2-year data from PARTNER B demonstrated significantly decreased mortality over medical management [2]. At 2 years, mortality in the standard therapy group was 68%, while it was 43% in the TAVR group [3]. Greater than 80% of the medical management group were treated with palliative balloon valvuloplasty, and 10% crossed over to TAVR, neither of which affected the marked survival benefit seen with TAVR. The cohort B patients who demonstrated the greatest survival benefit were those that had a low STS score (<5%) but were

© Springer International Publishing AG, part of Springer Nature 2018

A. C. Watkins et al., *Transcatheter Aortic Valve Replacement*, https://doi.org/10.1007/978-3-319-93396-2_2

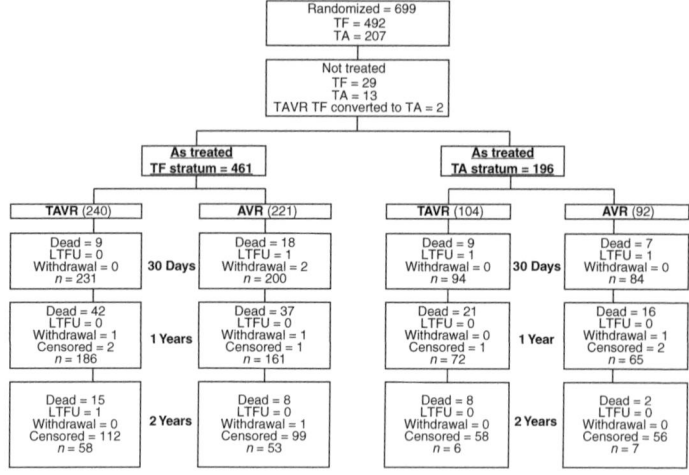

FIGURE 2.1 Design and results of the PARTNER (Placement of Aortic Transcatheter Valves) clinical trial. (JTCVS Volume 143, Issue 4, April 2012, Pages 832–843.e13)

inoperable secondary to porcelain aorta, chest radiation, or difficult redo surgery; at 5 years, all strata of patients regardless of STS risk score demonstrated benefit [4]. PARTNER B data revealed a significantly higher stroke rate in TAVR patients at 1 and 2 years, 13.8% in the TAVR group compared to 5.5% standard therapy at 2 years. The PARTNER B trial also demonstrated improvements in NYHA heart failure class and hospitalizations for heart failure compared to medically managed controls. PARTNER B patients demonstrated a significantly improved quality of life with multiple assessment tools [5]. PARTNER B proved TAVR to be the treatment of choice for inoperable patients.

The *PARTNER A* cohort consisted of 699 patients with STS risk >10% or surgeon assessment of mortality >15%, who were randomized to TAVR or SAVR. The cohort randomized to TAVR received the Edwards SAPIEN THV system. This study validated the non-inferiority of TAVR versus SAVR and allowed transcatheter therapies to be a viable, comparable option in high-risk patients. At 30 days, 1-year and 2-year mortality rates between the TAVR and surgical groups were not significantly different [1], with 33.9% mortality in the TAVR group and 35% in the SAVR group at 2 years [6]. Periprocedural stroke rate in PARTNER A was not significantly different among the two groups at 30 days. At 1 and 2 years, TAVR patients had a higher rate of stroke, 11.2% versus 6.5% in the SAVR patients at 2 years. The study also revealed increased vascular complications among the TAVR patients (11.6% vs 3.8%) and increased major bleeding episodes in the SAVR patients (29.5% vs 19%). Post-procedure renal failure, endocarditis, and new pacemaker placement were similar between the two groups. PARTNER A data illustrated increased post-procedure aortic insufficiency (AI) in the TAVR patients at 1 and 2 years, with 6.9% moderate to severe paravalvular AI in the TAVR group and 0.9% in the SAVR group at 2 years. The study went on to show that at 2 years, even a mild paravalvular leak was associated with increased mortality (HR 2.11) [6].

As the first and longest prospective, randomized clinical trial of TAVR therapy, the 5-year PARTNER A data extended earlier findings. At 5 years, mortality and rate of pacemaker implantation were similar, while TAVR was associated with increased vascular complications [4]. These studies identified both the lifesaving ability of TAVR technology and the common complications and limitations that advanced device development.

In parallel with the development of the SAPIEN system, the Medtronic CoreValve was examined in extreme (equivalent to inoperable in the PARTNER trials) and high-risk patients [7]. The high-risk trial randomized 795 patients to receive Medtronic's CoreValve or SAVR. Patients were deemed high risk if 2 cardiac surgeons and 1 interventional cardiologist agreed their risk of death or irreversible comorbidity was between 15% and 50% at 30 days. STS risk score was considered but not required for study inclusion. Both transfemoral and alternative access patients were included in the TAVR group prior to randomization. The average STS score of patients in the study was 7.4%. Expanding beyond the non-inferiority of TAVR therapy seen in the PARTNER

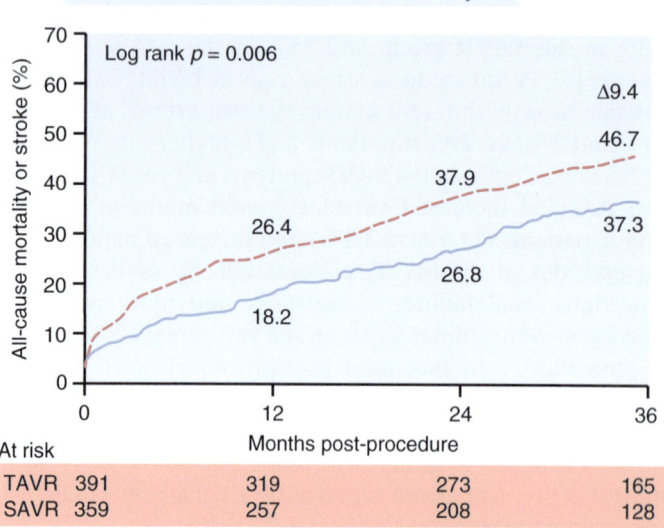

FIGURE 2.2 Improved results for TAVR compared to SAVR among high-risk patients receiving the CoreValve [10]

studies, 1- [8], 2- [9], and 3 [10]-year data from the trial demonstrated a *significantly improved survival* in TAVR compared with SAVR patients (Fig. 2.2).

Similar to PARTNER, this study found an increase in vascular injury (7% vs 2%) and decrease in life-threatening bleeding (18% vs 40%) among TAVR patients. At 2 years, the CoreValve saw a significant increase in stroke rate among the SAVR patients (11% vs 17%). It also revealed a decreased acute kidney injury (6% vs 15%) and significant pacemaker rate (26% vs 13%) compared to surgical therapy. At 3 years, the rate of mild perivalvular leak with the CoreValve was 51%, and moderate or greater leak was 6.8% (0% in the surgical arm) [10]. This study served to establish transcatheter therapy as the preferred treatment for high-risk severe aortic stenosis and the CoreValve as unique to the balloon-expandable devices with a different outcome profile.

Subsequent to the original PARTNER trial, the *PARTNER 2* randomized 2032 *intermediate-risk* patients, defined as an STS score between 4% and 8%, to the second-generation SAPIEN XT valve compared to SAVR. The primary endpoint of the study, death or disabling stroke, was similar among TAVR and SAVR patients, 19% vs 21%, at 2 years. Additionally, the TAVR group demonstrated increased vascular complications and perivalvular leak but decreased acute kidney injury, new-onset atrial fibrillation, and less severe bleeding when compared to the SAVR patients [11]. When outcomes of transfemoral TAVR and SAVR were compared, TAVR demonstrated a significantly lower rate of death or disabling stroke (HR 0.79). The newer generation SAPIEN 3 valve has also been compared to the SAVR arm of the PARTNER 2 trial in intermediate-risk patients. This observational study demonstrated both improved results with the SAPIEN 3 valve compared to the SAPIEN XT (7.4% mortality, 2% disabling stroke, and 2% moderate or greater perivalvular leak) as well as significant advantage of TAVR in a composite endpoint of death, stroke, or perivalvular leak when compared to surgery [12]. This study demonstrated the SAPIEN 3 valve to have a very low rate of moderate or severe perivalvular leak at 2%, which is improved compared to older generations and the CoreValve (5.3%) [13], but significantly higher than the AI rate following SAVR (0.5%). Both the SAPIEN 3 and CoreValve have significantly higher rates of mild AI compared to these studies that lead to the FDA approval of the SAPIEN 3 valve for use in intermediate-risk patients in August 2016. The PARTNER 2 trial highlights the most significant topic in TAVR clinical research: *Should TAVR therapy be used in younger, lower risk patients?* Current studies are examining TAVR results in low-risk (STS <3%) patients.

A significant theme of the PARTNER trials is the *inferior results among non-transfemoral access* patients [14]. In the early use of TAVR, transapical access via anterior left thoracotomy was the preferred alternative access for patients with prohibitively diseased femoral arteries. Transapical access patients in the high-risk PARTNER A trial had an elevated mortality (as compared to those in the transfemoral cohort) of 41% at 2 years. Patients in the transapical arm were considerably sicker than the transfemoral TAVR cohort, with increased history of stroke, peripheral vascular disease, atrial fibrillation, prior CABG, and porcelain aorta. In the intermediate-risk study, transthoracic (transapical or trans-aortic) access demonstrated a higher mortality (25%) at 2 years *compared to transfemoral or SAVR* [11]. For this rea-son, many programs have moved away from transapical access, instead of using subclavian, carotid, or even transcaval as second-line access for TAVR.

In addition to these large clinical trials done in the United States, there is a wealth of clinical information to be gleaned from individual company and country registries. The Society of Thoracic Surgeons and American College of Cardiology have developed the *Transcatheter Valve Therapy Registry* to follow outcomes of non-research TAVR and other transcath-eter procedures done in the United States. A recent report of TVT data on 26,414 TAVR patients illustrates a shifting risk profile of TAVR patients toward lower-risk patients. It reports an improved inhospital mortality (4.4%), vascular complication (4.2%), acute kidney injury (2.2%), and aortic insufficiency rate (26% any degree) in TAVR therapy. TVT Registry data also shows a stable stroke (2.2%) and proce-dural complication rate and increased need for permanent pacemakers (11%) among all TAVR patients [15].

References

1. Smith CR, Leon MB, Mack MJ, Miller DC, Moses JW, Svensson LG, Tuzcu EM, Webb JG, Fontana GP, Makkar RR, Williams M, Dewey T, Kapadia S, Babaliaros V, Thourani VH, Corso P, Pichard AD, Bavaria JE, Herrmann HC, Akin JJ, Anderson WN, Wang D, Pocock SJ, PARTNER Trial Investigators. Transcatheter versus surgical aortic-valve replacement in high-risk patients. N Engl J Med. 2011;364(23):2187–98.
2. Leon MB, Smith CR, Mack M, Miller DC, Moses JW, Svensson LG, Tuzcu EM, Webb JG, Fontana GP, Makkar RR, Brown DL,

Block PC, Guyton RA, Pichard AD, Bavaria JE, Herrmann HC, Douglas PS, Petersen JL, Akin JJ, Anderson WN, Wang D, Pocock S, PARTNER Trial Investigators. Transcatheter aortic-valve implantation for aortic stenosis in patients who cannot undergo surgery. N Engl J Med. 2010;363(17):1597–607.

3. Makkar RR, Fontana GP, Jilaihawi H, Kapadia S, Pichard AD, Douglas PS, Thourani VH, Babaliaros VC, Webb JG, Herrmann HC, Bavaria JE, Kodali S, Brown DL, Bowers B, Dewey TM, Svensson LG, Tuzcu M, Moses JW, Williams MR, Siegel RJ, Akin JJ, Anderson WN, Pocock S, Smith CR, Leon MB, PARTNER Trial Investigators. Transcatheter aortic-valve replacement for inoperable severe aortic stenosis. N Engl J Med. 2012;366(18):1696–704.

4. Mack MJ, Leon MB, Smith CR, Miller DC, Moses JW, Tuzcu EM, Webb JG, Douglas PS, Anderson WN, Blackstone EH, Kodali SK, Makkar RR, Fontana GP, Kapadia S, Bavaria J, Hahn RT, Thourani VH, Babaliaros V, Pichard A, Herrmann HC, Brown DL, Williams M, Akin J, Davidson MJ, Svensson LG. PARTNER 1 trial investigators. 5-year outcomes of transcatheter aortic valve replacement or surgical aortic valve replacement for high surgical risk patients with aortic stenosis (PARTNER 1): a randomized controlled trial. Lancet. 2015;385(9986):2477–84.

5. Reynolds MR, Magnuson EA, Wang K, Lei Y, Vilain K, Walczak J, Kodali SK, Lasala JM, O'Neill WW, Davidson CJ, Smith CR, Leon MB, Cohen DJ, PARTNER Trial Investigators. Cost-effectiveness of transcatheter aortic valve replacement compared with standard care among inoperable patients with severe aortic stenosis: results from the placement of aortic transcatheter valves (PARTNER) trial (cohort B). Circulation. 2012;125(9):1102–9.

6. Kodali SK, Williams MR, Smith CR, Svensson LG, Webb JG, Makkar RR, Fontana GP, Dewey TM, Thourani VH, Pichard AD, Fischbein M, Szeto WY, Lim S, Greason KL, Teirstein PS, Malaisrie SC, Douglas PS, Hahn RT, Whisenant B, Zajarias A, Wang D, Akin JJ, Anderson WN, Leon MB, PARTNER Trial Investigators. Two-year outcomes after transcatheter or surgical aortic-valve replacement. N Engl J Med. 2012;366(18):1686–95.

7. Popma JJ, Adams DH, Reardon MJ, Yakubov SJ, Kleiman NS, Heimansohn D, Hermiller J Jr, Hughes GC, Harrison JK, Coselli J, Diez J, Kafi A, Schreiber T, Gleason TG, Conte J, Buchbinder M, Deeb GM, Carabello B, Serruys PW, Chenoweth S, JK

O. CoreValve United States clinical investigators. Transcatheter aortic valve replacement using a self-expanding bioprosthesis in patients with severe aortic stenosis at extreme risk for surgery. J Am Coll Cardiol. 2014;63(19):1972–81.

8. Adams DH, Popma JJ, Reardon MJ, Yakubov SJ, Coselli JS, Deeb GM, Gleason TG, Buchbinder M, Hermiller J Jr, Kleiman NS, Chetcuti S, Heiser J, Merhi W, Zorn G, Tadros P, Robinson N, Petrossian G, Hughes GC, Harrison JK, Conte J, Maini B, Mumtaz M, Chenoweth S, JK O, U.S. CoreValve Clinical Investigators. Transcatheter aortic-valve replacement with a self-expanding prosthesis. N Engl J Med. 2014;370(19):1790–8.

9. Reardon MJ, Adams DH, Kleiman NS, Yakubov SJ, Coselli JS, Deeb GM, Gleason TG, Lee JS, Hermiller JB Jr, Chetcuti S, Heiser J, Merhi W, Zorn GL 3rd, Tadros P, Robinson N, Petrossian G, Hughes GC, Harrison JK, Maini B, Mumtaz M, Conte JV, Resar JR, Aharonian V, Pfeffer T, JK O, Qiao H, Popma JJ. 2-year outcomes in patients undergoing surgical or self-expanding Transcatheter aortic valve replacement. J Am Coll Cardiol. 2015;66(2):113–21.

10. Deeb GM, Reardon MJ, Chetcuti S, Patel HJ, Grossman PM, Yakubov SJ, Kleiman NS, Coselli JS, Gleason TG, Lee JS, Hermiller JB Jr, Heiser J, Merhi W, Zorn GL 3rd, Tadros P, Robinson N, Petrossian G, Hughes GC, Harrison JK, Maini B, Mumtaz M, Conte J, Resar J, Aharonian V, Pfeffer T, JK O, Qiao H, Adams DH, Popma JJ, CoreValve US Clinical Investigators. 3-year outcomes in high-risk patients who underwent surgical or Transcatheter aortic valve replacement. J Am Coll Cardiol. 2016;67(22):2565–74.

11. Leon MB, Smith CR, Mack MJ, Makkar RR, Svensson LG, Kodali SK, Thourani VH, Tuzcu EM, Miller DC, Herrmann HC, Doshi D, Cohen DJ, Pichard AD, Kapadia S, Dewey T, Babaliaros V, Szeto WY, Williams MR, Kereiakes D, Zajarias A, Greason KL, Whisenant BK, Hodson RW, Moses JW, Trento A, Brown DL, Fearon WF, Pibarot P, Hahn RT, Jaber WA, Anderson WN, Alu MC, Webb JG. PARTNER 2 investigators. Transcatheter or surgical aortic-valve replacement in intermediate-risk patients. N Engl J Med. 2016;374(17):1609–20.

12. Thourani VH, Kodali S, Makkar RR, Herrmann HC, Williams M, Babaliaros V, Smalling R, Lim S, Malaisrie SC, Kapadia S, Szeto WY, Greason KL, Kereiakes D, Ailawadi G, Whisenant BK, Devireddy C, Leipsic J, Hahn RT, Pibarot P, Weissman NJ, Jaber WA, Cohen DJ, Suri R, Tuzcu EM, Svensson LG,

Webb JG, Moses JW, Mack MJ, Miller DC, Smith CR, Alu MC, Parvataneni R, D'Agostino RB Jr, Leon MB. Transcatheter aortic valve replacement versus surgical valve replacement in intermediate-risk patients: a propensity score analysis. Lancet. 2016;387(10034):2218–25.

13. Reardon MJ, Van Mieghem NM, Popma JJ, Kleiman NS, Søndergaard L, Mumtaz M, Adams DH, Deeb GM, Maini B, Gada H, Chetcuti S, Gleason T, Heiser J, Lange R, Merhi W, JK O, Olsen PS, Piazza N, Williams M, Windecker S, Yakubov SJ, Grube E, Makkar R, Lee JS, Conte J, Vang E, Nguyen H, Chang Y, Mugglin AS, Serruys PW, Kappetein AP, SURTAVI Investigators. Surgical or Transcatheter aortic-valve replacement in intermediate-risk patients. N Engl J Med. 2017;376(14):1321–31.

14. Thourani VH, Forcillo J, Condado JF, Binongo JN, Babaliaros V, Lasanajak Y, Leshnower B, Devireddy C, Guyton R, Mavromatis K, Block P, Simone A, Keegan P, Stewart J, Tsai LL, Rajaei MH, Lerakis S, Sarin EL. Does a higher Society of Thoracic Surgeons score predict outcomes in Transfemoral and alternative access Transcatheter aortic valve replacement? Ann Thorac Surg. 2016;102(2):474–82.

15. Holmes DR Jr, Nishimura RA, Grover FL, Brindis RG, Carroll JD, Edwards FH, Peterson ED, Rumsfeld JS, Shahian DM, Thourani VH, Tuzcu EM, Vemulapalli S, Hewitt K, Michaels J, Fitzgerald S, Mack MJ. STS/ACC TVT registry. Annual outcomes with Transcatheter valve therapy: from the STS/ACC TVT registry. Ann Thorac Surg. 2016;101(2):789–800.

Chapter 3
Valves Available in the United States

SAPIEN 3

Derived from the SAPIEN THV used in the PARTNER trial, and the SAPIEN XT used in PARTNER 2A, the SAPIEN 3 (Fig. 3.1) valve is the most commonly used *balloon-expandable* transcatheter valve in the United States. It includes a cobalt-chromium frame and a trileaflet bovine pericardial valve. An improvement added to the SAPIEN 3 is a polyethylene tere-phthalate fabric cuff at the inflow of the valve, which has decreased the rate of perivalvular leak compared to earlier models [1] (www.Edwards.com).

The SAPIEN 3 Commander delivery system (Fig. 3.2) consists of a balloon catheter within a crimped valve. This is loaded within a flexible outer catheter. The delivery system includes a flex wheel (larger wheel in figure) which allows deflection of the tip of the catheter in the direction of the aorta as it goes up and over the arch. The ability to flex the delivery system allows aid in achieving a coplanar view of the valve prior to deployment. Features include a fine flex knob (red arrow) to aid in positioning and a lock to stably hold the balloon within the valve.

The Edwards system includes a *14 Fr* expandable eSheath (Fig. 3.3). The sheath features sealed additional plastic that expands to stretch up to 18 Fr as the valve passes through

© Springer International Publishing AG, part of Springer Nature 2018
A. C. Watkins et al., *Transcatheter Aortic Valve Replacement*, https://doi.org/10.1007/978-3-319-93396-2_3

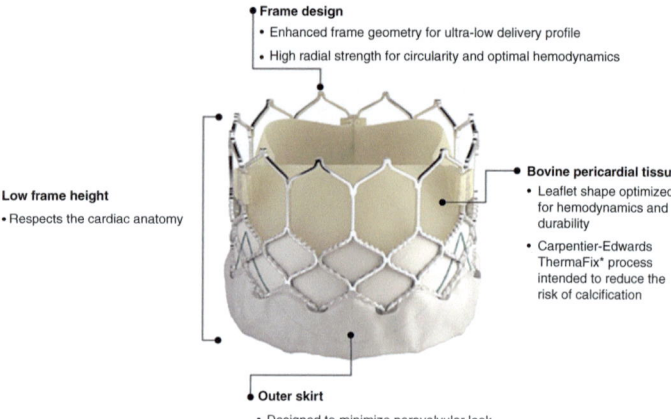

Frame design
• Enhanced frame geometry for ultra-low delivery profile
• High radial strength for circularity and optimal hemodynamics

Low frame height
• Respects the cardiac anatomy

Bovine pericardial tissue
• Leaflet shape optimized for hemodynamics and durability
• Carpentier-Edwards ThermaFix* process intended to reduce the risk of calcification

Outer skirt
• Designed to minimize paravalvular leak

FIGURE 3.1 The SAPIEN 3 TAVR valve by Edwards Lifesciences. (Used with permission from Edwards Lifesciences)

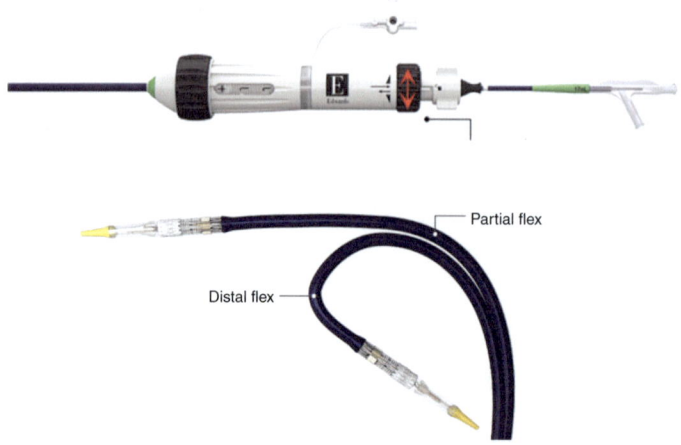

Partial flex

Distal flex

FIGURE 3.2 The SAPIEN 3 Commander delivery system. (Used with permission from Edwards Lifesciences)

then collapses back down to 14 Fr. It is recommended for use in femoral arteries <5.5 mm without significant calcific disease. For the size 29 valve, a 16 Fr sheath expands to 23 Fr to accommodate valve delivery through 6.0 mm vessels.

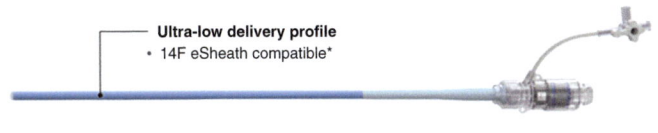

Ultra-low delivery profile
* 14F eSheath compatible*

SAPIEN 3 valve size	23 mm	26 mm	29 mm
Edwards eSheath introducer set	14F	14F	16F
Minimum access vessel diameter	5.5 mm	5.5 mm	6.0 mm

FIGURE 3.3 The Edwards system includes a 14 Fr expandable eSheath. (Used with permission from Edwards Lifesciences)

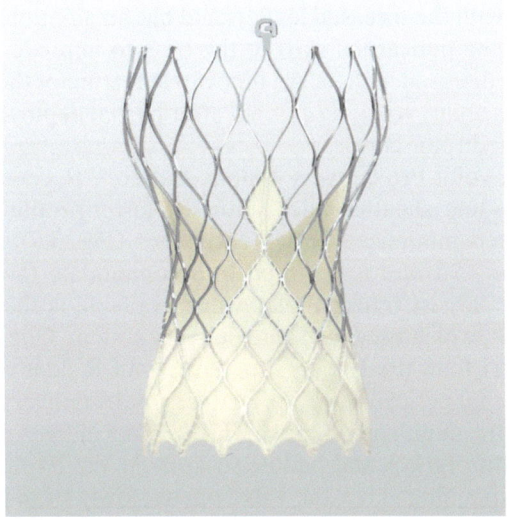

FIGURE 3.4 The Evolut Pro TAVR valve by Medtronic. (Used with permission from Medtronic)

EVOLUT Pro

The Evolut Pro (Medtronic, Minneapolis, MN) is the newest generation of the CoreValve which was used in the Medtronic high-risk trial (Fig. 3.4). It is the most commonly used *self-expanding* TAVR valve in the United States. It is a supra-annular, porcine tissue valve implanted within a nitinol frame. Porcine leaflets are preserved in alpha-amino oleic acid,

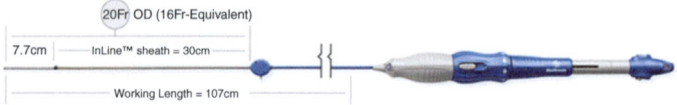

Figure 3.5 The Evolut Pro delivery system, EnVeo™ R. (Used with permission from Medtronic)

similar to surgical valves, to prevent calcium deposition. To improve upon the original CoreValve's perivalvular leak rate, the Evolut Pro valve shape is designed to increase the contact surface with the diseased leaflets and has an additional external porcine pericardial skirt at the base to improve the seal with the diseased leaflets. An innovative feature of the Evolut Pro is its ability to be *recaptured* after partial deployment [2] (www.medtronic.com).

The Evolut Pro delivery system, EnVeo™ R, consists of a 16 Fr in-line sheath, which allows a lower-profile arterial access and minimizes device exchanges (Fig. 3.5). Arterial diameter <5.5 *mm* is required to accommodate the Evolut Pro. The largest transcatheter valve available is the size 34 Evolut R, which uses the same delivery system. One generation older than the Evolut Pro, the Evolut R does not have the external pericardial wrap. Features of the delivery system include the deployment knob (white arrows in figure), recapture button (gray), and paddle sockets. As the Evolut Pro is a self-expanding valve, the valve opens slowly from the ventricular aspect in a 1:1 response from turning the deployment handle and self-centers within the native aortic valve. Annular contact is made initially with the non-coronary sinus, and as the valve base expands, contact is made with the left coronary sinus, securing the valve in place. At the most aortic aspect of the Evolut Pro valve, there are two paddles which hook into paddle sockets in the delivery system. This secure and straight connection between paddles and delivery system is critical to a smooth, well-positioned deployment, as the paddles are the last part of the valve to be released with full deployment.

TABLE 3.1 Additional TAVR valves available

Portico™ St Jude medical (St. Paul, MN) (used with permission from abbott.com)	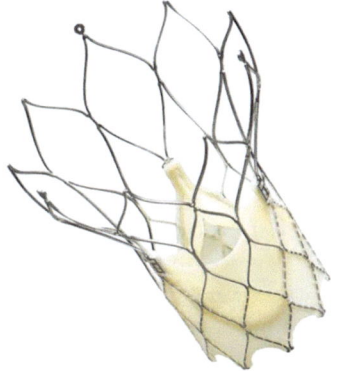
LOTUS edge™ Boston Scientific (Canton, MA)	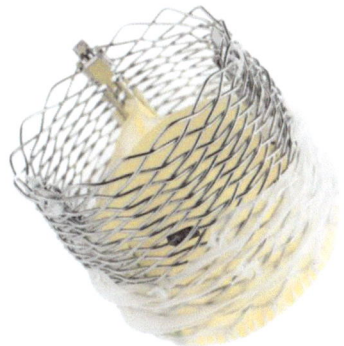
JenaValve™ JenaValve technologies (Irvine, CA)	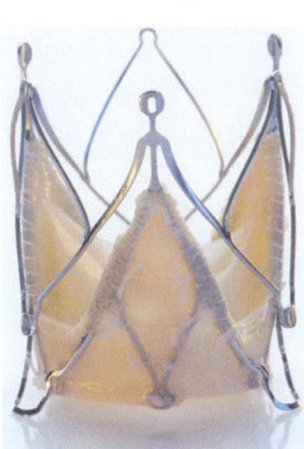

There are a variety of other transcatheter valves under investigation and approved for use in Europe. None are as heavily investigated or used as the SAPIEN and Evolut valves, but Table 3.1 illustrates a few that you may encounter in the literature or in future use. There are nearly a dozen more that have been tried in humans but are not widely used.

References

1. www.Edwards.com.
2. www.medtronic.com.

Chapter 4
Preoperative Evaluation: Indications and Risk Analysis

When evaluating a patient with AS, initial workup, definitions of severity, and indications for intervention will be the same for all AS patients as described in the *2014 AHA/ACC Guideline for the Management of Patients with Valvular Heart Disease* [1]. These most recent guidelines and a 2017 update include the recommendations for transcatheter procedures below [2]:

Class I Recommendations

1. Surgical AVR is recommended for patients with severe and low- or intermediate-risk AS, regardless of symptoms.
2. Surgical AVR or TAVR is recommended for high-risk patients with symptomatic, severe AS depending on patient procedural risk, anatomy, or preference.
3. TAVR is recommended for prohibitive-risk patients with symptomatic, severe AS who are predictive to live 1 year.
4. For high-risk patients with AS, a multidisciplinary heart valve team should collaborate to provide the best recommendation.

© Springer International Publishing AG, part of Springer Nature 2018
A. C. Watkins et al., *Transcatheter Aortic Valve Replacement*, https://doi.org/10.1007/978-3-319-93396-2_4

Class IIa Recommendations

1. TAVR is a reasonable alternative to SAVR in intermediate-risk patients with symptomatic, severe AS depending on patient procedural risk, anatomy, or preference.

Class IIb Recommendations

1. Balloon valvuloplasty may serve as a bridge to either SAVR or TAVR in severely symptomatic AS patients.

Class III Recommendation: No Benefit

1. TAVR is not recommended in patients with significant comorbidity that would preclude benefit from AVR.

These recommendations can be summarized in protocol below from the *2017 AHA/ACC Focused Update of the 2014 AHA/ACC Guideline for the Management of Patients with Valvular Heart Disease* [2] (Fig. 4.1).

Considerations of both medical comorbidity and surgical anatomy will direct a SAVR or TAVR recommendation.

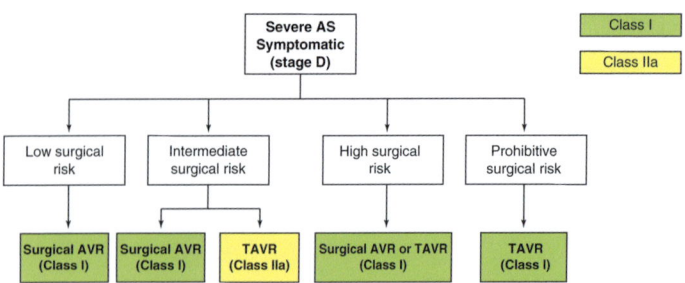

FIGURE 4.1 Choice of TAVR versus surgical AVR in the patient with severe symptomatic AS (JACC Jul 2017, 70 (2) 252–289). AS indicates aortic stenosis; AVR aortic valve replacement, TAVR transcatheter aortic value replacement

There are a few key points to notice the above recommendations. A patient must be symptomatic to receive a TAVR. Neither AS therapy is appropriate for a patient without expectation of benefit from AS correction or with limited life expectancy secondary to other comorbid conditions. The majority of work defining safety and use in TAVR has been done using *The Society of Thoracic Surgeons (STS) risk calculator*. This score will risk stratify patients, <4% as low risk, 4–8% as intermediate risk, and >8% as high risk, for either SAVR or TAVR. Although TAVR is currently under investigation for use in low-risk patients, SAVR is currently the recommended therapy for patients with an STS score <4% without precluding factors. Based on the above recommendations, in symptomatic, low-risk AS patients, SAVR is a class I and TAVR a class IIa recommendation. Additional considerations when deciding treatment modality in any risk profile include concurrent diseases requiring repair, such as coronary, aneurysmal, or other valve disease. The STS score captures a good degree of comorbidity, but doesn't account for porcelain aorta, liver dysfunction, pulmonary hypertension, radiation exposure, mobility, use of home oxygen, or frailty. Additionally, recurrent publications examining the observed mortality rate following SAVR in comparison with risk predicted by the STS score find better than expected mortality. For these reasons, STS score cannot be the sole determinant of therapy modality. Like any cardiac operation, surgical planning will be nuanced and individual.

More quantitative measures of *frailty* have been developed and applied to TAVR evaluation, including assessments of weight loss, weakness, exhaustion, low activity, and slow walk speed. Patients gain a point for each substandard result in each of the 5 categories, with a score ≥3 signifying a patient as frail. Unintentional weight loss ≥5 kg in 12 months gains a point. Exhaustion and low activity are positive responses to specific survey questions. Weakness is assessed with grip strength, and slowness is assessed with a 5-meter walk test, both with specific cutoffs for sex and size. Frail patients have worse outcomes with any surgical procedure and should be considered TAVR.

Comorbidity is an important consideration when planning a TAVR procedure, and recent data can give insight into outcomes of TAVR in the setting of various comorbidities. Unfortunately, many common comorbidities were excluded from the initial prospective trials of TAVR. Any type of AVR in patients with end-stage renal disease (*ESRD*) poses increased risk of complication or poor outcome. Multiple studies demonstrate that as GFR goes down, mortality goes up, among both TAVR and SAVR patients [3, 4]. Results comparing TAVR to SAVR retrospectively present equivocal outcomes in ESRD patients [5]. Chronic kidney disease (*CKD*) engenders risk in both TAVR due to contrast exposure resulting in CIN and SAVR due to cardiopulmonary bypass exposure. Although not compared in any prospective studies, studies report a low incidence of permanent renal failure in CKD patients following TAVR [6] but mixed results as to the benefit of TAVR or SAVR in CKD patients [3, 7].

Other comorbid conditions that require consideration include *COPD*, which is not uncommon among severe AS patients. Home O_2 use is a very poor prognostic factor for both TAVR and SAVR [8]. There is evidence that pulmonary function can improve following TAVR [9]. With moderate or severe COPD, TAVR with conscious sedation is preferable to SAVR which has an increased risk of tracheostomy and prolonged course [10]. Advanced *cirrhosis* is known to be a very poor predictor of outcome following cardiac surgery; there is increasing use of TAVR in patients with liver disease. Retrospective analysis suggests a mortality of 6.7% in both SAVR and TAVR patients with liver disease but fewer complications with TAVR [11]. *Reoperation* is a risk for increased morbidity or mortality with subsequent cardiac surgery. Reports examining the CoreValve high-risk trial retrospectively showed better outcomes for TAVR patients with prior CABG [12]. Additionally, while heart failure increases the procedural risk of TAVR, the majority of patients with *reduced ejection fraction* will see improvement following

TAVR [13]. All risk factors require careful analysis and balance of risk and benefits. These comorbidities may become less relevant as TVAR therapy is extended toward lower-risk patients.

Contraindications

A clear contraindication to TAVR is *infectious endocarditis*, as stenting infection into the aortic annulus, left ventricular outflow tract (LVOT), or aortic root would be disastrous (Table 4.1). Suspicion of aortic valve endocarditis should be referred for surgery. Native *aortic insufficiency* (AI) without aortic stenosis is also a current contraindication to TAVR; the annular calcium present in degenerative AS is required for the device to form an anchor in the annulus. However AI in the setting of severe AS or a degenerated bioprosthetic valve can be successfully treated with TAVR. There are case reports and small case series of successful use of TAVR for AI, generally in patients at prohibitive risk for surgery. Results tend to be inferior to TAVR for AS with a higher incidence of valve embolism, secondary interventions,

TABLE 4.1 Contraindications to TAVR or SAVR

Contraindications to TAVR	Contraindications to SAVR
Infective endocarditis	Prohibitive reoperative anatomy
Bacteremia	Prior chest radiation
Aortic insufficiency without stenosis	Porcelain aorta
Prohibitive annular size	Prior sternal wound infection
No aortic access	Inability to be anticoagulated
Intracardiac mass or thrombus	
Mobile aortic atheroma	
Inability to be anticoagulated	

residual AI, and death [14]. The JenaValve™ (JenaValve Technologies, Irvine, CA) is the leading transcatheter devices being investigated for the use of native aortic valve insufficiency. Anatomic restrains of TAVR are prohibitive annular sizes, extensive peripheral atherosclerosis prohibiting access for TAVR. Other exclusions include intracardiac mass or thrombus, inability to be anticoagulated for the procedure, and significant, mobile aortic atheroma. Contraindications to SAVR include difficult redo sternotomies often secondary to known dense adhesions, excessive chest radiation, prior deep sternal wound infection or mediastinitis complicating potential redo surgery, or CAB grafts adherent to sternotomy. Patients with a *porcelain aorta* have few surgical options and are preferentially referred for TAVR. All of these factors must be evaluated and considered when deciding between a SAVR or TAVR recommendation.

Understanding the risks of each procedure and how those would effect a particular patient is important in determining treatment modality. In general, TAVR carries an increased risk of perivalvular leak/AI (2–3% of patients will have moderate to severe PVL versus under 1% for SAVR in a similar risk patient population) and vascular complications, while SAVR has an increased risk of major bleeding, AKI, and new AF.

Bicuspid Aortic Valve

Although excluded from the majority of clinical trials in TAVR, bicuspid disease is not a contraindication for TAVR. Bicuspid valves tend to have bulky calcifications and a higher point of coaptation compared to tricuspid valves. An asymmetric annulus and tendency for aortic dilation may also complicate TAVR for bicuspid valves. Early-generation devices demonstrated TAVR therapy to be feasible and safe in bicuspid AV disease but with a higher rate of mortality and perivalvular leak, particularly with self-expanding valves [15, 16]. First-generation devices also exhibited an increased rate of annular injury and a second valve implantation with used in the bicuspid aortic valve. With newer-generation devices, procedural complications have decreased, and perivalvular leak has improved from 8.5–14.7 to 0–2.7% [17, 18]. Currently, all studies examining TAVR in bicuspid AV are retrospective. Two recent studies using new-generation balloon-expandable and self-expanding devices suggest a similar rate of procedural success, moderate or severe perivalvular leak, and operative and 30-day and 2-year mortality among bicuspid and tricuspid TAVR patients [16, 19]. Another series with 51 patients demonstrated no moderate or severe perivalvular leak in bicuspid aortic valves following TAVR with the SAPIEN 3; however the rate of mild AI is reported as high as 37% [20]. Given mild perivalvular leak was associated with higher long-term mortality in the PARTNERS data, this may prove to be a risk with TAVR for bicuspid disease. Permanent pacemaker implantation following TAVR for bicuspid valves ranges from 15 to 26% [16, 21], which is higher than currently reported for SAPIEN 3 in tricuspid valves. The additional anatomic complexity of bicuspid aortic valve disease requires additional planning (described below) and risk considerations for TAVR but does not preclude successful therapy. Patients with any concomitant aneurysmal disease should be treated with surgery, as subsequent ascending aorta or aortic root repair will be more difficult following TAVR. As the most common congenital cardiac disease, effecting up to 2% of the population, TAVR for bicuspid AV disease will likely grow and evolve during your practice.

Valve-in-Valve

Transcatheter therapy is used to treat failed surgical bioprosthetic aortic valve with valve-in-valve procedures. The lifespan on a bioprosthetic surgical aortic valve approaches 15–20 years but is often less in younger patients [22]. Elderly patients undergoing SAVR years ago present with valve failure due to recurrent AS and AI. Much older than at their initial operation, many of these patients have the comorbidities and contraindications mentioned above prohibiting redo SAVR. Valve-in-valve procedures should be offered to patients with bioprosthetic valve disease when the risks of open surgery outweigh the risk of TAVR if anatomy allows. *Transesophageal echocardiogram* is required preoperatively, not only to aid in sizing but also to confirm any AI is not perivalvular and can be corrected by a valve-in-valve TAVR. It is important to rule out patient prosthesis mismatch prior to procedures for AS, as increasing gradients with mobile leaflets maybe secondary to increasing patient size [23]. Most current knowledge of valve-in-valve outcomes derives from a Global Valve-in-Valve Registry that started in 2010 [24, 25]. Data from this registry demonstrated a 7.6% 30-day mortality, a 2% stroke rate, and a 16.8% 1-year mortality. Risks for 1-year mortality were valve sizes less than or equal to 21 and *restenosis* rather than AI as the mode of prosthesis failure. There is an increased rate of *coronary obstruction* complications in valve-in-valve procedures at 3.5%. Mean aortic valve gradient is generally higher following valve-in-valve than native TAVR, with 28% in the global registry having a mean gradient >20 mmHg. Residual high valve gradients are a more substantial problem than the smaller surgical valve size. This data also revealed that valve-in-valve TAVR with self-expanding prosthesis had significantly increased moderate AI versus balloon-expandable valves (8.9 vs 2.4%) and that balloon-expandable valves had higher mean valve gradients (9.7 vs 7.3 mmHg) and more patients with gradients >20 mmHg [25]. It is unknown whether the higher mean gradients seen in valve-in-valve TAVR will limit their durability. Retrospective attempts at comparing valve-in-valve TAVR with reoperative SAVR have shown similar mortality [26] but with small patient numbers.

Generally, compared to first-time TAVR, valve-in-valve procedures result in fewer perivalvular leaks, annular rupture, or permanent pacemaker placement but increased device malposition, coronary obstruction, and post-procedure valve gradients [23]. Avoidance of malpositioning or coronary obstruction comes from comprehensive understanding of the structure of the surgical valve, which will be integrated through

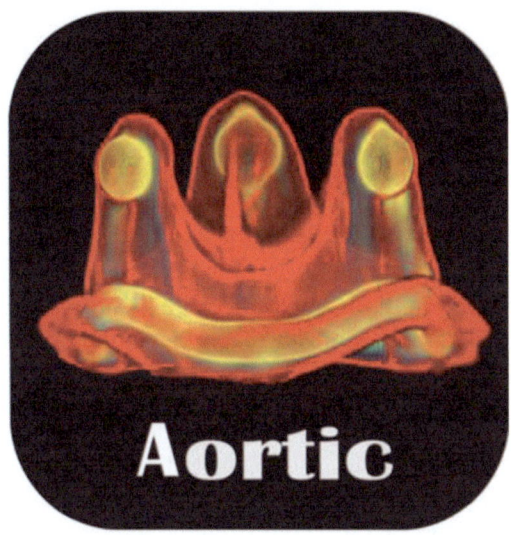

FIGURE. 4.2 Valve-in-valve app. (Used with permission from www. ubqo.com/viv)

the surgical report, perioperative TEE, CT, and fluoroscopy. The fluoroscopic details of each surgical valve as well as a useful starting point in sizing (discussed below) and positioning are available in an app (Fig. 4.2) designed by English cardiac surgeon, Mr. Vinnie Bapat.

While this app can offer assistance, there is no replacement for measuring the annulus or inner diameter of a surgical valve yourself (described below). Surgical valves with the leaflets attached to the external surface of the frame, such as the Mitroflow (Sorin) or Trifecta (St. Jude), are particularly prone to coronary obstruction and should cautiously considered for valve-in-valve procedures. Likewise, stentless prostheses and homografts would be very challenging and should generally be avoided.

A description of placing a larger TAVR valve in a failing surgical bioprosthetic valve by "cracking" the surgical valve with a non-compliant balloon dilatation catheter has been reported [27]. This technique is relatively new, and more data will be required to ensure that this method is safe. For patients at risk for bioprosthetic leaflet occlusion of the coronary arteries, methods to pre-wire the low coronary and stent post-deployment if necessary have been used. This technique also is in the early stages of experience, and there is a paucity of literature at the time of publication of this manual.

At times the choice of SAVR or TAVR will be patient directed. Patients often have preconceptions about which therapy they want. This will affect their motivation during recovery. Through knowledgeable recommendations and patient education, you can offer the optimal therapy, but you may need to keep in mind patient preference. In all instances, the decision between TAVR and SAVR is best made by a *dedicated heart team*, including cardiologist, interventionalists, and surgeons. CMS currently mandates that a cardiologist and two surgeons examine the patient and their imaging before offering a TAVR procedure. Joining this aortic valve heart team will not only help establish your TAVR expertise but also introduce you to many SAVR patients as well.

References

1. Nishimura RA, Otto CM, Bonow RO, Carabello BA, Erwin JP 3rd, Guyton RA, O'Gara PT, Ruiz CE, Skubas NJ, Sorajja P, Sundt TM 3rd, Thomas JD, ACC/AHA Task Force Members. 2014 AHA/ACC guideline for the management of patients with valvular heart disease: a report of the American College of Cardiology/American Heart Association task force on practice guidelines. Circulation. 2014;129(23):e521–643.
2. Nishimura RA, Otto CM, Bonow RO, Carabello BA, Erwin JP 3rd, Fleisher LA, Jneid H, Mack MJ, McLeod CJ, O'Gara PT, Rigolin VH, Sundt TM 3rd, Thompson A. 2017 AHA/ACC focused update of the 2014 AHA/ACC guideline for the management of patients with valvular heart disease: a report of the American College of Cardiology/American Heart Association task force on clinical practice guidelines. J Am Coll Cardiol. 2017;70(2):252–89.

3. Nguyen TC, Babaliaros VC, Razavi SA, Kilgo PD, Guyton RA, Devireddy CM, Shults CC, Mavromatis K, Kanitkar M, Block P, Lerakis S, Thourani VH. Impact of varying degrees of renal dysfunction on transcatheter and surgical aortic valve replacement. J Thorac Cardiovasc Surg. 2013;146(6):1399–406.

4. Codner P, Levi A, Gargiulo G, Praz F, Hayashida K, Watanabe Y, Mylotte D, Debry N, Barbanti M, Lefèvre T, Modine T, Bosmans J, Windecker S, Barbash I, Sinning JM, Nickenig G, Barsheshet A, Kornowski R. Impact of renal dysfunction on results of transcatheter aortic valve replacement outcomes in a large multicenter cohort. Am J Cardiol. 2016;118(12):1888–96.

5. Szerlip M, Kim RJ, Adeniyi T, Thourani V, Babaliaros V, Bavaria J, Herrmann HC, Anwaruddin S, Makkar R, Chakravarty T, Rovin J, Creighton D, Miller DC, Baio K, Walsh E, Katinic J, Letterer R, Trautman L, Herbert M, Farkas R, Rudolph J, Brown D, Holper EM, Mack M. The outcomes of transcatheter aortic valve replacement in a cohort of patients with end-stage renal disease. Catheter Cardiovasc Interv. 2016;87(7):1314–21.

6. Goebel N, Baumbach H, Ahad S, Voehringer M, Hill S, Albert M, Franke UF. Transcatheter aortic valve replacement: does kidney function affect outcome? Ann Thorac Surg. 2013;96(2):507–12.

7. D'Errigo P, Moretti C, D'Ascenzo F, Rosato S, Biancari F, Barbanti M, Santini F, Ranucci M, Miceli A, Tamburino C, Onorati F, Santoro G, Grossi C, Fusco D, Seccareccia F. OBSERVANT Research Group. Transcatheter aortic valve implantation versus surgical aortic valve replacement for severe aortic stenosis in patients with chronic kidney disease stages 3b to 5. Ann Thorac Surg. 2016;102(2):540–7. https://doi.org/10.1016/j.athoracsur.2016.01.109. Epub 2016 Apr 26

8. Dvir D, Waksman R, Barbash IM, Kodali SK, Svensson LG, Tuzcu EM, Xu K, Minha S, Alu MC, Szeto WY, Thourani VH, Makkar R, Kapadia S, Satler LF, Webb JG, Leon MB, Pichard AD. Outcomes of patients with chronic lung disease and severe aortic stenosis treated with transcatheter versus surgical aortic valve replacement or standard therapy: insights from the PARTNER trial (placement of AoRTic TraNscathetER valve). J Am Coll Cardiol. 2014;63(3):269–79.

9. Gilmore RC, Thourani VH, Jensen HA, Condado J, Binongo JN, Sarin EL, Devireddy CM, Leshnower B, Mavromatis K, Syed A, Guyton RA, Block PC, Simone A, Keegan P, Stewart J, Rajaei M, Kaebnick B, Lerakis S, Babaliaros VC. Transcatheter aortic valve replacement results in improvement of pulmonary func-

tion in patients with severe aortic stenosis. Ann Thorac Surg. 2015;100(6):2167–73.

10. Hyman MC, Vemulapalli S, Szeto WY, Stebbins A, Patel PA, Matsouaka RA, Herrmann HC, Anwaruddin S, Kobayashi T, Desai ND, Vallabhajosyula P, McCarthy FH, Li R, Bavaria JE, Giri J. Conscious sedation versus general anesthesia for transcatheter aortic valve replacement: insights from the National Cardiovascular Data Registry Society of thoracic surgeons/ American College of Cardiology Transcatheter Valve Therapy Registry. Circulation. 2017;136(22):2132–40.

11. Thakkar B, Patel A, Mohamad B, Patel NJ, Bhatt P, Bhimani R, Patel A, Arora S, Savani C, Solanki S, Sonani R, Patel S, Patel N, Deshmukh A, Mohamad T, Grines C, Cleman M, Mangi A, Forrest J, Badheka AO. Transcatheter aortic valve replacement versus surgical aortic valve replacement in patients with cirrhosis. Catheter Cardiovasc Interv. 2016;87(5):955–62.

12. Conte JV, Gleason TG, Resar JR, Adams DH, Deeb GM, Popma JJ, Hughes GC, Zorn GL, Reardon MJ. Transcatheter or surgical aortic valve replacement in patients with prior coronary artery bypass grafting. Ann Thorac Surg. 2016;101(1):72–9.

13. Dauerman HL, Reardon MJ, Popma JJ, Little SH, Cavalcante JL, Adams DH, Kleiman NS, Oh JK. Early recovery of left ventricular systolic function after CoreValve transcatheter aortic valve replacement. Circ Cardiovasc Interv. 2016;9(6):1–10.

14. Sawaya FJ, Deutsch MA, Seiffert M, Yoon SH, Codner P, Wickramarachchi U, Latib A, Petronio AS, Rodés-Cabau J, Taramasso M, Spaziano M, Bosmans J, Biasco L, Mylotte D, Savontaus M, Gheeraert P, Chan J, Jørgensen TH, Sievert H, Mocetti M, Lefèvre T, Maisano F, Mangieri A, Hildick-Smith D, Kornowski R, Makkar R, Bleiziffer S, Søndergaard L, De Backer O. Safety and efficacy of transcatheter aortic valve replacement in the treatment of pure aortic regurgitation in native valves and failing surgical bioprostheses: results from an international registry study. JACC Cardiovasc Interv. 2017;10(10):1048–56.

15. Kochman J, Huczek Z, Scisło P, Dabrowski M, Chmielak Z, Szymański P, Witkowski A, Parma R, Ochala A, Chodór P, Wilczek K, Reczuch KW, Kubler P, Rymuza B, Kołtowski L, Scibisz A, Wilimski R, Grube E, Opolski G. Comparison of one- and 12-month outcomes of transcatheter aortic valve replacement in patients with severely stenotic bicuspid versus tricuspid aortic valves (results from a multicenter registry). Am J Cardiol. 2014;114(5):757–62.

16. Yoon SH, Bleiziffer S, De Backer O, Delgado V, Arai T, Ziegelmueller J, Barbanti M, Sharma R, Perlman GY, Khalique OK, Holy EW, Saraf S, Deuschl F, Fujita B, Ruile P, Neumann FJ, Pache G, Takahashi M, Kaneko H, Schmidt T, Ohno Y, Schofer N, Kong WKF, Tay E, Sugiyama D, Kawamori H, Maeno Y, Abramowitz Y, Chakravarty T, Nakamura M, Kuwata S, Yong G, Kao HL, Lee M, Kim HS, Modine T, Wong SC, Bedgoni F, Testa L, Teiger E, Butter C, Ensminger SM, Schaefer U, Dvir D, Blanke P, Leipsic J, Nietlispach F, Abdel-Wahab M, Chevalier B, Tamburino C, Hildick-Smith D, Whisenant BK, Park SJ, Colombo A, Latib A, Kodali SK, Bax JJ, Søndergaard L, Webb JG, Lefèvre T, Leon MB, Makkar R. Outcomes in transcatheter aortic valve replacement for bicuspid versus tricuspid aortic valve stenosis. J Am Coll Cardiol. 2017;69(21):2579–89.

17. Yoon SH, Sharma R, Chakravarty T, Kawamori H, Maeno Y, Miyasaka M, Nomura T, Ochiai T, Israr S, Rami T, Nakamura M, Chen W, Makkar RR. Clinical outcomes and prognostic factors of transcatheter aortic valve implantation in bicuspid aortic valve patients. Ann Cardiothorac Surg. 2017;6(5):463–72.

18. Yoon SH, Lefèvre T, Ahn JM, Perlman GY, Dvir D, Latib A, Barbanti M, Deuschl F, De Backer O, Blanke P, Modine T, Pache G, Neumann FJ, Ruile P, Arai T, Ohno Y, Kaneko H, Tay E, Schofer N, Holy EW, Luk NHV, Yong G, Lu Q, Kong WKF, Hon J, Kao HL, Lee M, Yin WH, Park DW, Kang SJ, Lee SW, Kim YH, Lee CW, Park SW, Kim HS, Butter C, Khalique OK, Schaefer U, Nietlispach F, Kodali SK, Leon MB, Ye J, Chevalier B, Leipsic J, Delgado V, Bax JJ, Tamburino C, Colombo A, Søndergaard L, Webb JG, Park SJ. Transcatheter aortic valve replacement with early- and new-generation devices in bicuspid aortic valve stenosis. J Am Coll Cardiol. 2016;68(11):1195–205.

19. Sannino A, Cedars A, Stoler RC, Szerlip M, Mack MJ, Grayburn PA. Comparison of efficacy and safety of transcatheter aortic valve implantation in patients with bicuspid versus tricuspid aortic valves. Am J Cardiol. 2017;120(9):1601–6.

20. Perlman GY, Blanke P, Dvir D, Pache G, Modine T, Barbanti M, Holy EW, Treede H, Ruile P, Neumann FJ, Gandolfo C, Saia F, Tamburino C, Mak G, Thompson C, Wood D, Leipsic J, Webb JG. Bicuspid aortic valve stenosis. Favorable Early Outcomes With a Next-Generation Transcatheter Heart Valve in a Multicenter Study JACC Cardiovasc Interv. 2016;9(8):817–24.

21. Jilaihawi H, Chen M, Webb J, Himbert D, Ruiz CE, Rodés-Cabau J, Pache G, Colombo A, Nickenig G, Lee M, Tamburino

C, Sievert H, Abramowitz Y, Tarantini G, Alqoofi F, Chakravarty T, Kashif M, Takahashi N, Kazuno Y, Maeno Y, Kawamori H, Chieffo A, Blanke P, Dvir D, Ribeiro HB, Feng Y, Zhao ZG, Sinning JM, Kliger C, Giustino G, Pajerski B, Imme S, Grube E, Leipsic J, Vahanian A, Michev I, Jelnin V, Latib A, Cheng W, Makkar R. A bicuspid aortic valve imaging classification for the TAVR era. JACC Cardiovasc Imaging. 2016;9(10):1145–58.

22. Foroutan F, Guyatt GH, O'Brien K, Bain E, Stein M, Bhagra S, Sit D, Kamran R, Chang Y, Devji T, Mir H, Manja V, Schofield T, Siemieniuk RA, Agoritsas T, Bagur R, Otto CM, Vandvik PO. Prognosis after surgical replacement with a bioprosthetic aortic valve in patients with severe symptomatic aortic stenosis: systematic review of observational studies. BMJ. 2016;354:i5065.

23. Dvir D, Barbanti M, Tan J, Webb JG. Transcatheter aortic valve-in-valve implantation for patients with degenerative surgical bioprosthetic valves. Curr Probl Cardiol. 2014;39(1):7–27.

24. Dvir D, Webb J, Brecker S, Bleiziffer S, Hildick-Smith D, Colombo A, Descoutures F, Hengstenberg C, Moat NE, Bekeredjian R, Napodano M, Testa L, Lefevre T, Guetta V, Nissen H, Hernández JM, Roy D, Teles RC, Segev A, Dumonteil N, Fiorina C, Gotzmann M, Tchetche D, Abdel-Wahab M, De Marco F, Baumbach A, Laborde JC, Kornowski R. Transcatheter aortic valve replacement for degenerative bioprosthetic surgical valves: results from the global valve-in-valve registry. Circulation. 2012;126(19):2335–44.

25. Dvir D, Webb JG, Bleiziffer S, Pasic M, Waksman R, Kodali S, Barbanti M, Latib A, Schaefer U, Rodés-Cabau J, Treede H, Piazza N, Hildick-Smith D, Himbert D, Walther T, Hengstenberg C, Nissen H, Bekeredjian R, Presbitero P, Ferrari E, Segev A, de Weger A, Windecker S, Moat NE, Napodano M, Wilbring M, Cerillo AG, Brecker S, Tchetche D, Lefèvre T, De Marco F, Fiorina C, Petronio AS, Teles RC, Testa L, Laborde JC, Leon MB, Kornowski R. Valve-in-valve international data registry investigators. Transcatheter aortic valve implantation in failed bioprosthetic surgical valves. JAMA. 2014;312(2):162–70.

26. Wilbring M, Tugtekin SM, Alexiou K, Simonis G, Matschke K, Kappert U. Transapical transcatheter aortic valve implantation vs conventional aortic valve replacement in high-risk patients with previous cardiac surgery: a propensity-score analysis. Eur J Cardiothorac Surg. 2013;44(1):42–7.

27. Chhatriwalla AK, Allen KB, Saxon JT, Cohen DJ, Aggarwal S, Hart AJ, Baron SJ, Dvir D, Borkon AM. Bioprosthetic valve

fracture improves the hemodynamic results of valve-in-valve transcatheter aortic valve replacement. Circ Cardiovasc Interv. 2017;10(7). pii: e005216

Chapter 5
Preoperative Imaging

Necessary to the preoperative planning of any TAVR procedure are as follows:

1. Cardiac-gated CTA with femoral vessel runoff
2. High-quality transthoracic echo or transesophageal echo
3. Evaluation for coronary disease/angiogram

The cardiac-gated CTA is used to determine critical measurements needed to size and place the valve. Obtaining optimal retrospective gated imaging is key to making adequate measurements—close collaboration with the radiologist at a site new to TAVR imaging is a must. Review of the CTA with 3-D modeling software and determination of measurements should be done in consultation with the interventional cardiologist, cardiac surgeon and device company representative. Different institutions will use different reconstruction software; familiarizing yourself with the version available to you and being able to confirm sizing will help you understand and be involved in process. There are differences in the measuring of structures based on which valve you are using. Edwards products determine the valve size based on AV area, while Medtronic products determine the size on valve perimeter. Both products take measurements in systole.

The measurements needed for TAVR procedural planning include:

© Springer International Publishing AG, part of Springer Nature 2018
A. C. Watkins et al., *Transcatheter Aortic Valve Replacement*,
https://doi.org/10.1007/978-3-319-93396-2_5

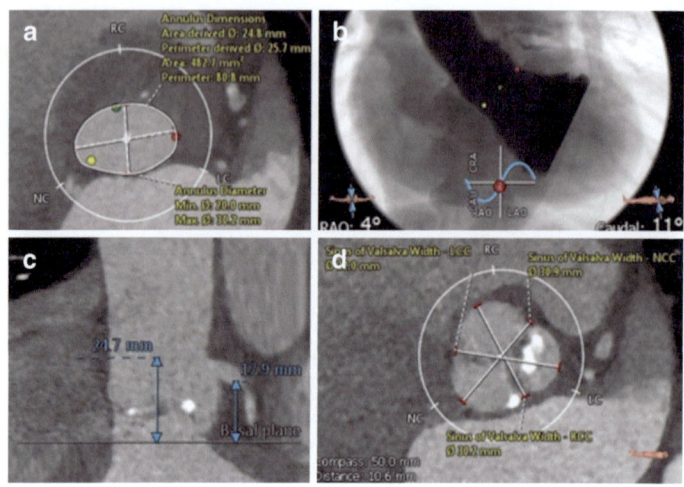

FIGURE 5.1 Pre-TAVR CTA. (**a**) Annular size. (**b**) Deployment angle. (**c**) Sinus and coronary heights. (**d**) Sinus of Valsalva size

1. Annular size (area and perimeter)
2. Sinuses of Valsalva
3. Coronary heights
4. Sinotubular junction
5. Mid-ascending aorta
6. Left ventricular outflow tract
7. Coplanar delivery angle

The AV *annulus* is measured at the nadir of each sinus of Valsalva (Fig. 5.1). Its elliptical shape must be determined at this position by careful outlining with reconstruction software. The *sinuses of Valsalva* are measured at the point in which the sinuses are the widest. Each of the three sinuses is measured from the widest point of the sinus to the opposing valve commissure. This figure illustrates some of the measurements needed on a commonly used software system, 3mensio™: (Pie Medical, the Netherlands).

The *coronary height* needed to safely position a transcatheter valve is generally *1 cm*. It is measured from the nadir of the sinus to the inferior aspect of the coronary ostia. When evaluating coronary heights, this measurement must be related to the size of the sinuses of Valsalva, as larger sinuses will allow increased room between your valve and coronary ostia as any given coronary height. Generally coronary heights of 1 cm and sinuses over 3 cm will not cause coronary obstruction by a transcatheter valve. Coronary heights less than 1 cm may still accommodate a TAVR when the sinuses of Valsalva are large. When coronary obstruction is a concern, alterations in approach to deployment are crucial (described below) but may also lead the team to consider a recapturable valve.

Left ventricular outflow tract (LVOT) and *sinotubular junction* (STJ) height also need to be quantified. The LVOT is measured 3 mm below the annulus; an LVOT diameter of <2 cm should raise concern for possible device embolization. An STJ height less than 2 cm should raise concern for a small root and possible coronary obstruction. When evaluating the annulus on CTA, it will be necessary to determine the *coplanar axis* at which the three nadirs of the annulus are in the same flat plane. This projection angle will provide the view at which the device should be deployed. By marking the annulus at the nadir of each sinus, this plane can be determined by reconstruction software. It will also be confirmed on the intra-procedural root angiogram.

In addition to aortic measurements, the CTA is necessary to note the locations of *heavy calcium deposition* or *tortuosity* throughout the vasculature (Fig. 5.2). This will be critical to both device selection and procedural planning. Heavy calcium anywhere in the thoracic aorta will increase the risk of periprocedural stroke. Circumferential calcification in the vasculature poses a risk of vascular injury. Heavy annular or *LVOT calcium* will increase the risks of stroke, annular rupture, and perivalvular leak. A tortuous or hairpin turn in the aortic arch poses a risk for aortic, annular, or ventricular injury and may lead the team to consider an alternative access. A *horizontal heart* is an angle between the perpendicular plane of the AV annulus and a horizontal reference line less than 30°. Making device delivery and positioning

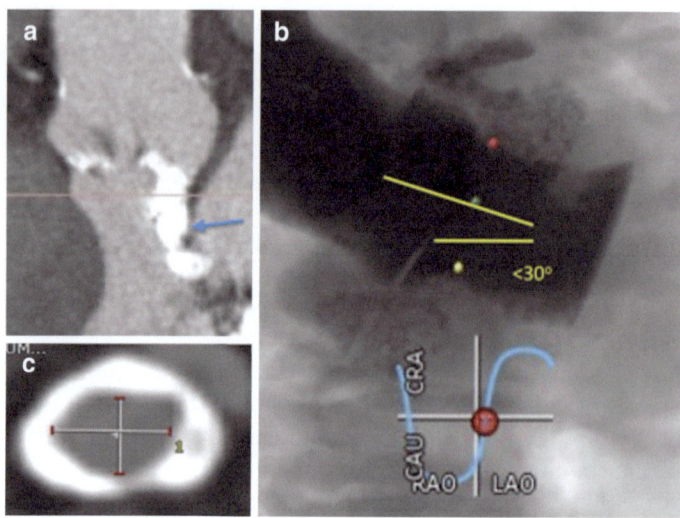

FIGURE 5.2 CTA findings predicting catastrophe. (**a**) Left ventricular outflow tract calcium. (**b**) Horizontal heart. (**c**) Circumferential calcium in access vessels

increasingly difficult, a horizontal heart can predispose to ventricular or aortic injury.

The abdominal and pelvic portions of the CTA will determine if the patient has vasculature compatible with transfemoral access. By choosing the centerline of the iliac and femoral vessels and outlining the vessels in multiple places, reconstruction can determine the size of the entire iliofemoral vasculature. The femoral vessels should be measured at the femoral head and above the bifurcation of the superficial femoral and profunda arteries. Averaging repeat measurement will increase your accuracy. The entire iliofemoral vasculature should be examined for tortuosity, calcium deposition, and aneurysm. A heavily calcified or tortuous iliac or femoral artery should be avoided for device access. It is important to remember the recommended *minimum femoral artery size* for each delivery system is based on a *non-calcified* artery.

In patients with *chronic renal insufficiency*, we have had success using a pigtail catheter placed in the main pulmonary artery to reduce contrast dose. Immediately prior to pre-TAVR CT, a 5Fr pigtail catheter is advanced from the femoral vein to the main pulmonary artery. Rather than 120 cc of contrast used in CT angiogram via a peripheral IV, we are able to obtain adequate imaging with 25 cc contrast via the pulmonary artery catheter [1].

Preoperative echocardiogram will confirm the degree of AS, demonstrate leaflet anatomy and degree of calcification, presence of any AI, other possible valvular dysfunction as well as estimate ventricular function. It will be important to not only exclude pathologies that might also give a high measured gradient, such as septal hypertrophy, but also to identify cases of severe AS without clearly elevated gradients. With long-standing severe AS, hypertrophy and eventual myocardial fibrosis will result in clinical heart failure and a depressed ejection fraction (EF), termed *low-flow, low-gradient AS*. These patients have calcified, stenotic valves but not the ventricular function to mount gradients across the AV typically classified as severe. In this situation, a *dobutamine stress echocardiogram* will be necessary to demonstrate increased stroke volume, EF, and AV gradients, confirming your diagnosis. If dobutamine causes an increase in EF but not AV gradient, the patient's systolic heart failure is much more significant than any outflow obstruction, termed pseudo-AS. If gradients increase with inotropy, this suggests myocardial reserve sufficient to benefit from AVR. If stroke volume increased by *>20%*, mean AV gradient increased to *>40 mmHg,* and AV area remains *<1.0 cm2*, the patient has true severe AS. Low EF patients exhibiting increased stroke volume and AV gradient on dobutamine echo, without coronary artery disease and with a mean gradient greater than 20 mmHg at rest, have been shown to have the best prognosis with SAVR and therefore are likely to benefit most from TAVR as well [2, 3]. Additional complicated scenarios include low-flow, low-gradient severe aortic stenosis without contractile reserve; low-flow, low-gradient preserved ejection fraction aortic stenosis; and normal-flow, low-gradient preserved ejection fraction aortic stenosis. These entities are complicated, less well understood than high-gradient aortic stenosis, and require careful consideration.

Coronary workup with *angiogram* should be considered in all patients. In patients being considered for surgery or TAVR, coronary angiogram will not only exclude the need for CABG or PCI but also give information as to the height and shape of the coronary takeoffs. Cardiac catheterization will also give more reliable measurements of AV gradient than will echocardiogram. Cardiac-gated CTA to evaluate coronary disease is a secondary option. In particularly elderly patients with underlying renal insufficiency in whom the primary concern is heart failure, a heart team may decide to forgo coronary angiography. Access to the coronary arteries after TAVR valve deployment can be more difficult and should be taken into consideration.

Bicuspid Aortic Valve

The key to successful treatment lies in high-quality imaging, accurate sizing, and a detailed understanding of the bicuspid anatomy. There are conflicting reports regarding the success of TAVR for bicuspid disease depending on Sievers type [4]. Risks for inaccurate sizing and perivalvular leak include annular eccentricity, fused raphe with bulky calcium, asymmetric valve cusps, and left ventricular outflow tract calcium [5]. Multi-slice CT provides a more reliable assessment of bicuspid valve anatomy than echo and has been shown to improve outcomes with bicuspid AV [6, 7]. CT assessment begins as it does for tricuspid valves with identification of the annulus at the nadir of the sinuses of Valsalva. Sizing for bicuspid AV disease has been described using annular area and perimeter as done for tricuspid valves as well as sizing a few millimeters above the annulus at the commissural level. In Sievers type 0, there are only 2 sinuses of Valsalva to provide a nadir point at which the annulus can be measured. In this situation, an examination of the prosthesis landing zone just a few millimeters below the annulus can add an addition estimate of size. CT evaluation of bicuspid valves must include *identification of the raphe, commissures, and leaflets*. Examination of these structures for heavy calcium deposits, severe asymmetry, or thickened, long raphe may help identify bicuspid anatomy at high risk for perivalvular leak or procedural complications [5]. Do not forget to look for aortic aneurysms!

Valve-in-Valve

Valve-in-valve cases require careful planning to find a transcatheter valve that will fit well within their previous tissue valve. Determined by CT scan, the true internal diameter and height of the bioprosthetic valve will determine if and what transcatheter valve will work. Visualizing and understanding the fluoroscopic appearance of both the surgical and transcatheter valves will help determine the ideal placement of a valve-in-valve TAVR. The size of a surgical valve as stated by the manufacturer is generally the outer diameter of the prosthesis. For valve-in-valve TAVR, the *inner diameter* should be considered the "annular size" to base TAVR sizing (Fig. 5.3). Additional considerations include the height of the leaflets and stents or posts. These measurements, along with sinus sizes and coronary height, can help to avoid coronary obstruction. Additionally, the height at which the surgical valve is implanted will vary, ranging from intra- to supra-annular, and needs to be taken into account to avoid coronary obstruction. Any anatomy with *low coronary ostia, narrow sinuses of Valsalva, tall leaflets, or high supra-annular position* should raise concerns for coronary occlusion with valve-in-valve TAVR. Given that bioprosthetic valves are often not as heavily calcified as native valves making leaflets difficult to see on fluoroscopy, intraoperative TEE-assisted positioning can be helpful in valve-in-valve TAVR [8].

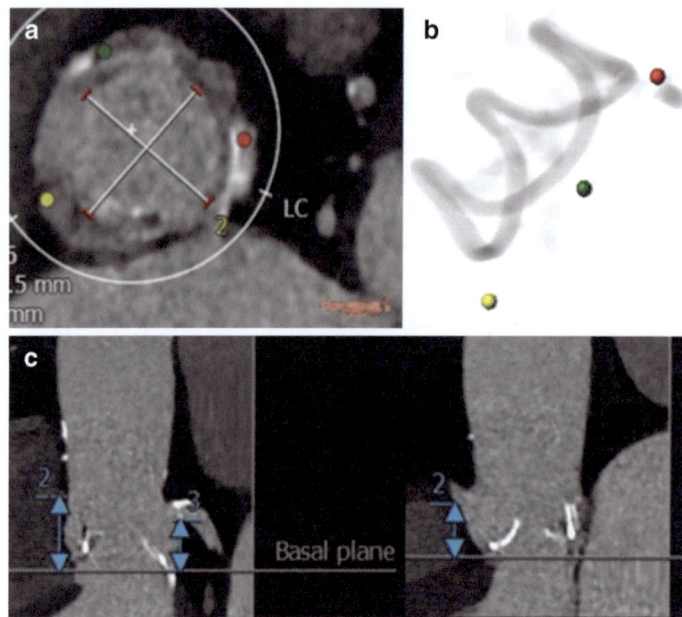

FIGURE 5.3 Pre-TAVR imaging for valve-in-valve. (**a**) Inner diameter "annular" measurement. (**b**) Deployment angle. (**c**) Coronary heights

References

1. Chahal DS, Ginsberg E, Kligerman SJ, Jeudy J, Seliger S, Meeks A, Lee T, Gupta A. TCT-661 low contrast dose CTA for TAVR evaluation using central pulmonary artery catheter. J Am Coll Cardiol. 2015;66(15_S):B271.
2. Chrissoheris M, Ziakas A, Chalapas A, Chadjimiltiades S, Styliades I, Karvounis C, Nikolaou I, Spargias K. Acute invasive hemodynamic effects of transcatheter aortic valve replacement. J Heart Valve Dis. 2016;25(2):162–72.
3. Holmes DR Jr, Mack MJ, Kaul S, Agnihotri A, Alexander KP, Bailey SR, Calhoon JH, Carabello BA, Desai MY, Edwards FH, Francis GS, Gardner TJ, Kappetein AP, Linderbaum JA, Mukherjee C, Mukherjee D, Otto CM, Ruiz CE, Sacco RL, Smith D, Thomas JD. 2012 ACCF/AATS/SCAI/STS expert consensus

document on transcatheter aortic valve replacement. J Am Coll Cardiol. 2012;59(13):1200–54.

4. Yousef A, Simard T, Webb J, Rodés-Cabau J, Costopoulos C, Kochman J, Hernández-Garcia JM, Chiam PT, Welsh RC, Wijeysundera HC, García E, Ribeiro HB, Latib A, Huczek Z, Shanks M, Testa L, Farkouh ME, Dvir D, Velianou JL, Lam BK, Pourdjabbar A, Glover C, Hibbert B, Labinaz M. Transcatheter aortic valve implantation in patients with bicuspid aortic valve: a patient level multi-center analysis. Int J Cardiol. 2015;189:282–8.

5. Popma JJ, Ramadan R. CT imaging of bicuspid aortic valve disease for TAVR. JACC Cardiovasc Imaging. 2016;9(10):1159–63.

6. Kong WK, Regeer MV, Ng AC, McCormack L, Poh KK, Yeo TC, Shanks M, Parent S, Enache R, Popescu BA, Yip JW, Ma L, Kamperidis V, van der Velde ET, Mertens B, Ajmone Marsan N, Delgado V, Bax JJ. Sex differences in phenotypes of bicuspid aortic valve and aortopathy: insights from a large multicenter, international registry. Circ Cardiovasc Imaging. 2017;10(3). pii: e005155

7. Mylotte D, Lefevre T, Søndergaard L, Watanabe Y, Modine T, Dvir D, Bosmans J, Tchetche D, Kornowski R, Sinning JM, Thériault-Lauzier P, O'Sullivan CJ, Barbanti M, Debry N, Buithieu J, Codner P, Dorfmeister M, Martucci G, Nickenig G, Wenaweser P, Tamburino C, Grube E, Webb JG, Windecker S, Lange R, Piazza N. Transcatheter aortic valve replacement in bicuspid aortic valve disease. J Am Coll Cardiol. 2014;64(22):2330–9.

8. Dvir D, Barbanti M, Tan J, Webb JG. Transcatheter aortic valve-in-valve implantation for patients with degenerative surgical bioprosthetic valves. Curr Probl Cardiol. 2014;39(1):7–27.

Chapter 6
Self-Expanding Versus Balloon-Expandable Devices

In addition to individual patient factors, the selection of a device must consider the anatomy of the LV outflow tract, annulus, root, and location of the coronary arteries. Considerations in valve type including annular size, degree of calcification, and arterial access will be relevant to valve choice. The figure below outlines some of the considerations we use at our institution. These are theoretical considerations as there is no substantial data to support either valve types in specific clinical scenarios. The vast majority of work comparing the valve types is retrospective and shows no difference in survival [1–3]. There has been one randomized, prospective clinical trial comparing the valve types, which demonstrated similar outcomes, except for increased perivalvular leak and pacemaker placement with self-expanding valves [4].

Trends to keep in mind when selecting a valve are slightly increased rate of perivalvular leak and permanent pacemaker requirement with self-expanding valves, and the risk of annular rupture, while infrequent, is higher with balloon-expandable valves. Self-expanding valves demonstrate lower valve gradients. It is not known if a small difference in gradient affects long-term durability. The Evolut Pro can be used for larger valve areas and offers the unique feature of recapturability. Any TAVR in which positioning is anticipated to be precarious, such as with low coronary arteries, the

© Springer International Publishing AG, part of Springer Nature 2018

A. C. Watkins et al., *Transcatheter Aortic Valve Replacement*, https://doi.org/10.1007/978-3-319-93396-2_6

Small Valve	
Large Valve	
Annular Ca2+/Risk rupture	
Pre-BAV/tight valve	
Pre-existing Pacemaker	
Tortuous vascular access	
Bicuspid Aortic Valve	
Horizontal deployment angle	
Heart failure	
Low Coronaries	
Valve-in-valve	

EvolutePro	Lower gradients
EvolutePro	Size 34
EvolutePro	Lower radial force
Sapien 3	Higher radial force
EvolutePro	No new pacemaker risk
Sapien 3	Flex delivery
Anatomy dependent	Higher radial force vs. recapturable
Sapien 3	Flex delivery
Sapien 3	Lower pacemaker risk
EvolutePro	Repositionable
EvolutePro	Lower gradients, recapturable

CONSIDERATIONS IN TAVR DEVICE SELECTION

recapturability of an Evolut Pro may be attractive. With significant calcifications, a self-expanding valve may decrease the risk of annular rupture; however, there will be an accompanying increased risk of perivalvular leak. The risks of annular rupture secondary to annular or LVOT calcium need to be weighed against the risks of perivalvular leak and permanent pacemaker. In valves that are so stenotic, a balloon valvuloplasty (BAV) is required prior to valve implantation in order to accommodate the passing of the device through the valve; a SAPIEN 3 can be advocated. A BAV already exposes the patient to the risks of balloon-expansion, which would be compounded with the risk of self-expanding valves. In patients that already have a pacemaker, a self-expanding valve risk profile may be preferred. However, in heart failure patients, in whom loss of their native sinus rhythm would be detrimental, a balloon-expandable valve might be the better choice. The flex feature of the SAPIEN 3 delivery system makes it well-suited for patients with a hairpin-shaped aorta, a horizontal heart, or tortuous access vasculature [2]. These are some of the possible concerns, but ultimately, the best criteria for selecting a valve may be surgeon preference.

References

1. Watanabe Y, Hayashida K, Yamamoto M, Mouillet G, Chevalier B, Oguri A, Dubois-Rande JL, Morice MC, Teiger E, Lefèvre T. Transfemoral aortic valve implantation in patients with an annulus dimension suitable for either the Edwards valve or the CoreValve. Am J Cardiol. 2013;112(5):707–13.
2. Wijeysundera HC, Qiu F, Koh M, Prasad TJ, Cantor WJ, Cheema A, Chu MW, Czarnecki A, Feindel C, Fremes SE, Kingsbury K, Natarajan MK, Peterson M, Ruel M, Strauss B, Ko DT. Comparison of outcomes of balloon-expandable versus self-expandable Transcatheter heart valves for severe aortic stenosis. Am J Cardiol. 2017;119(7):1094–9.
3. Tarantini G, Purita PAM, D'Onofrio A, Fraccaro C, Frigo AC, D'Amico G, Fovino LN, Martin M, Cardaioli F, Badawy MRA, Napodano M, Gerosa G, Iliceto S. Long-term outcomes and prosthesis performance after transcatheter aortic valve replacement: results of self-expandable and balloon-expandable transcatheter heart valves. Ann Cardiothorac Surg. 2017;6(5):473–83.
4. Abdel-Wahab M, Mehilli J, Frerker C, Neumann FJ, Kurz T, Tölg R, Zachow D, Guerra E, Massberg S, Schäfer U, El-Mawardy M, Richardt G, investigators CHOICE. Comparison of balloon-expandable vs self-expandable valves in patients undergoing transcatheter aortic valve replacement: the CHOICE randomized clinical trial. JAMA. 2014;311(15):1503–14.

Chapter 7
Valve Sizing

Annular sizing for the SAPIEN 3 valve is measured in systole on the cardiac CT scan and based on annular area. Edwards Lifesciences provides information regarding the degree of over- or undersizing for each valve size and annular area (Fig. 7.1). If between sizes, the volume in the balloon can be adjusted to 1–2 cc. oversizing can lead to annular rupture, pacemaker requirement, or coronary obstruction, while undersizing can lead to perivalvular leak or device embolization. If annular size is on the boarder of two sizes and the anatomy exhibits high annular or LVOT calcium, low coronaries, or a small sinotubular junctions, pick the smaller size. Oversizing >20% poses significant risk for annular rupture and is not recommended [1]. When choosing to oversize, significant annular or LVOT calcium should be considered.

While sizing for the CoreValve was done in diastole, the Evolut Pro valve is now based on annular perimeter in systole. The size of the sinuses of Valsalva, sinotubular junction, and the coronary heights should also be considered when choosing a valve size (Fig. 7.2). When on the border between sizes, a smaller root should receive the smaller valve size to avoid coronary obstruction.

When there is significant asymmetric valve calcium, a bicuspid valve, or CT-determined annular size boarder two valve sizes, intra-procedural *balloon sizing* can give insight to the true size of the annulus. Done with valvuloplasty balloon,

A. C. Watkins et al., *Transcatheter Aortic Valve Replacement*, https://doi.org/10.1007/978-3-319-93396-2_7

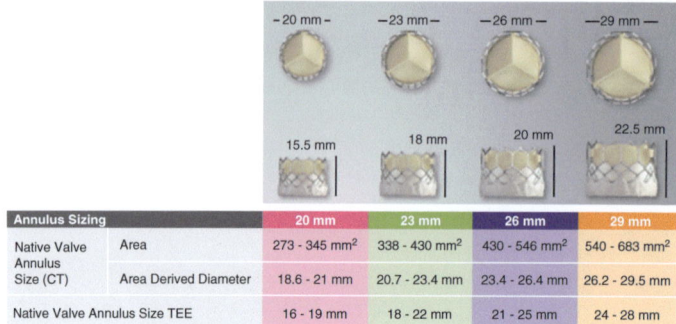

Annulus Sizing		20 mm	23 mm	26 mm	29 mm
Native Valve Annulus Size (CT)	Area	273 - 345 mm²	338 - 430 mm²	430 - 546 mm²	540 - 683 mm²
	Area Derived Diameter	18.6 - 21 mm	20.7 - 23.4 mm	23.4 - 26.4 mm	26.2 - 29.5 mm
Native Valve Annulus Size TEE		16 - 19 mm	18 - 22 mm	21 - 25 mm	24 - 28 mm

FIGURE 7.1 Edwards Lifesciences SAPIEN 3 annular sizing reference. (Used with permission from Edwards Lifesciences)

Evolut™ TAVR system
Valve size selection criteria per msct

	Valve size	Aortic annulus measurements		Sinus of valsalva diameter	Sinus of valsalva height
		Diameter	Perimeter		
Evolut™ PRO and Evolut™ R valves	23 mm	17†/18–20 mm	53.4†/56.5–62.8 mm	≥ 25 mm	≥15 mm
	26 mm	20–23 mm	62.8–72.3 mm	≥ 27 mm	≥15 mm
	29 mm	23–26 mm	72.3–81.7 mm	≥ 29 mm	≥15 mm
Evolut™ R valves	34 mm	26–30 mm	81.7–94.2 mm	≥ 31 mm	≥16 mm

FIGURE 7.2 Medtronic's Evolut™ annular sizing reference. (Used with permission from Medtronic). †Measurement for TAV-in-SAV only. Note: The dimensions of SAVs can change in vivo requiring multiple considerations for the physician to make and informed decision of what appropriate Evolut TAVR valve size to use for TAV-in-SAV. These considerations include identification of the SAV, determination of the manufacturer's inside diameter, CT estimated measurement of the SAV's annulus diameter and patient specifics as outlined in the Best Practices

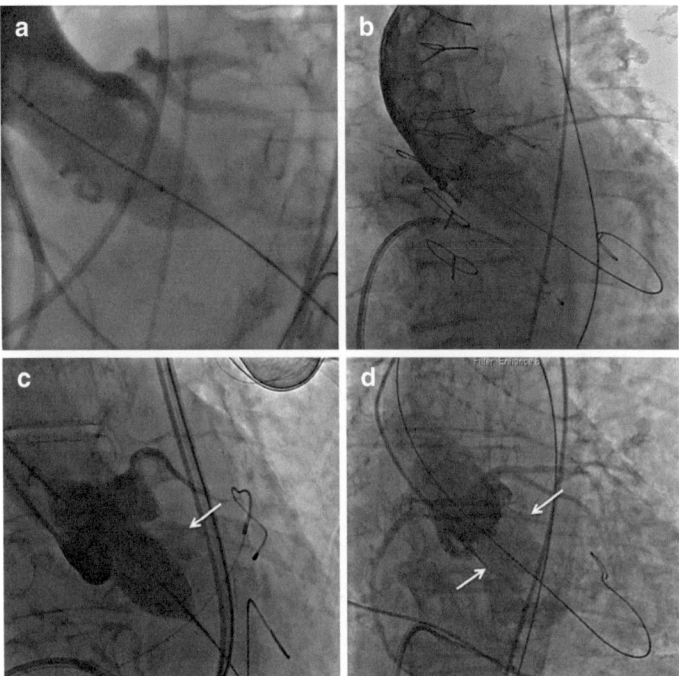

FIGURE 7.3 Intra-procedural balloon sizing of aortic annulus. Transannular balloon inflation with simultaneous aortogram while observing for absence (**a**, **b**) or presence (**c**, **d**) of contrast around the balloon into the ventricle [2]

such as a Z-MED™ (B. Braun Medical, Bethlehem, PA), aortic root angiography is taken with a balloon inflated in the annulus to examine for regurgitation around the balloon. If no leak around the balloon, a valve size 10% larger than the valvuloplasty balloon is generally recommended [2] (Fig. 7.3).

References

1. Binder RK, Rodés-Cabau J, Wood DA, Mok M, Leipsic J, De Larochellière R, Toggweiler S, Dumont E, Freeman M, Willson AB, Webb JG. Transcatheter aortic valve replacement with the

SAPIEN 3: a new balloon-expandable transcatheter heart valve. JACC Cardiovasc Interv. 2013;6(3):293–300.

2. Condado JF, Lerakis S, Stewart J, Jensen H, Henry TS, Ko SM, Stillman A, Rajaei MH, Mavromatis K, Devireddy C, Sarin E, Leshnower B, Guyton R, Kaebnick B, Thourani VH, Block PC, Babaliaros V. Balloon versus computed tomography sizing of the aortic annulus for Transcatheter aortic valve replacement and the impact of left ventricular outflow tract calcification and morphology on sizing. J Invasive Cardiol. 2016;28(7):295–304.

Chapter 8
Aortic Access Planning and Procedures

Percutaneous transfemoral access is known to be less morbid than alternative approaches but can be difficult in a patient with peripheral vascular disease. It is preferred because of its speed of use, interventionists' experience, and effective closure devices. The size of the delivery system of each valve has been approved for a certain diameter femoral artery (Table 8.1). It is important to remember this is a minimum size in a normal, non-atherosclerotic vessel. With significant calcium deposits or tortuosities, you will require a larger vessel.

Vascular complications with transfemoral access occur in 6% with current generation devices [1, 2]. Complications to watch for include iliac or femoral artery rupture or dissection, critical stenosis of the femoral artery created by your arteriotomy closure, or peripheral embolization of atherosclerotic debris. If iliofemoral vascular disease prohibits transfemoral access, as it does in 10–15% of TAVR patients, there are a variety of alternative access sites to consider.

Transapical

Transapical access is an option for patients with systemically obstructing atherosclerosis. Most all patients can tolerate a small anterior thoracotomy. Extremely poor pulmonary

© Springer International Publishing AG, part of Springer Nature 2018
A. C. Watkins et al., *Transcatheter Aortic Valve Replacement*,
https://doi.org/10.1007/978-3-319-93396-2_8

TABLE 8.1 Arterial access sizing for various TAVR devices

Valve	Valve size	Delivery system size (Fr)	Minimal femoral artery size (mm)
SAPIEN 3	20	14	5.5
	23	14	5.5
	26	14	5.5
	29	16	6.0
Evolut R	23	14	5.0
	26	14	5.0
	29	14	5.0
	34	16	5.5
Evolut Pro	23	16	5.5
	26	16	5.5
	29	16	5.5

function and frailty are general contraindications to transapical access. Post-procedure *outcomes are significantly worse* with transapical, likely secondary to the overall preoperative patient risk profile. For this reason, transapical access use is decreasing in many centers. Transapical access requires the apex to be located by CT and/or handheld echo prior to incision. This insures that the axis for delivery of the valve runs parallel to the septum. Additionally, direct ascending aortic access can be done through median sternotomy or upper hemi-sternotomy. This again exposes the patient to the pain and pulmonary insult of a sternotomy and would not be an option in the setting of porcelain aorta [3, 4]. Remember that the aortic puncture must be distal in the ascending aorta to allow for the action of the delivery system.

1. Position the patient supine with a roll under the left chest.
2. Localize the cardiac apex on CT scan. Looking in all three planes can help identify the rib space and laterally of the apex. Confirm the position of the apex on fluoroscopy prior to incision. Ensuring your thoracotomy is directly

over the apex will allow a small thoracotomy and straight-forward procedure.

3. A 4–6 cm anterolateral thoracotomy using a soft tissue retractor ± a Finochietto or Tuffier retractor generally provides good exposure.

4. The pericardium is opened and stay sutures help to expose the apex. On palpation, there is usually an indentation or dimple that can be felt at the true apex. The exact apex can again be confirmed under TEE while manually pok-ing your intended target. Mark the best near-apex loca-tion with a marking pen which avoids the LAD and other small coronary branches. It is preferred if the area for sutures is relatively free of epicardial fat. In the case of reoperation or significant pericardial adhesions, the peri-cardium can be minimally opened or left intact. Apical sutures may be placed through both the pericardium and myocardium. While this strengthens the buttress of the sutures, it risks inadvertent injury to coronary branches

5. Two perpendicularly interlocked and pledgeted, 3.0 pro-lines on *MH needles* are placed around the intended access site and snared with rammel tourniquets. We rec-ommend using large pledgets. The MH needles enable near-full thickness bites in the myocardium. The needle must be passed atraumatically to reduce the risk of tearing.

6. Accessing the left ventricle with a needle and *guidewire* under TEE guidance. The wire is passed along the septum and through the aortic valve. This ensures the correct tra-jectory for the sheath and device and avoids injury to the mitral apparatus or ventricle.

7. A 6Fr sheath is inserted through the apex over a soft wire. Through any catheter (pigtail or AL1), exchange the guidewire for a stiffer, Lunderquist wire. Confirm that your wire is not through the mitral apparatus.

8. Depending on your valve type and size, introduce a 14–20Fr sheath through the apex and 4–5 cm into the left ventricle. Edwards Lifesciences makes a shorter Certitude™ sheath for use in transthoracic TAVR. Although the Evolut Pro comes with an in-line sheath, we recommend placing the

device through a sheath 1 Fr size larger than the device and retracting the in-line sheath. Dedicate one team member to *hold the sheath* in place. Ventricular pressure will tend to expel the sheath even if secured to the skin.

9. Prepare and *reverse load* the transcatheter valve with the aortic end of the valve toward the nosecone.

10. Deploy the transcatheter valve (positioning and deployment described in Chapter 10).

11. Remove the sheath with the patient in Trendelenburg position. Reintroduce the sheath dilator so that the sheath can be slowly and stably removed. One person removes the sheath over the wire, while two others synch down on the tourniquets. If sutures are stable and hemostatic, the wire can then be removed and the sutures sequentially tied. If either suture appears to be inadequate for hemostatic repair of the apex, the sheath can be reintroduced and addition of pledgeted, purse-string sutures can be placed. Rapidly pace the heart to reduce LV pressure during the tie down.

12. Close the thoracotomy in the standard fashion leaving a pericardial and left pleural drain. Losing approximating the pericardium provides reinforcing tissue between your apical access site and the chest wall. Local nerve block is helpful.

Subclavian

The preferred secondary access site at our institution is the subclavian artery, which has been shown to have outcomes similar to transfemoral procedures [5, 6]. The subclavian artery can be accessed either through an anterior subclavicular incision or percutaneously. Noting the *depth* of the subclavian on preoperative CT can help decide the approach (Fig. 8.1). A deeper artery will pose a more acute angle for device delivery. We prefer surgical exposure; the subclavian artery can be access directly or via an anastomosed 8.0 mm graft. While placing a surgical graft may lengthen the procedure, it can

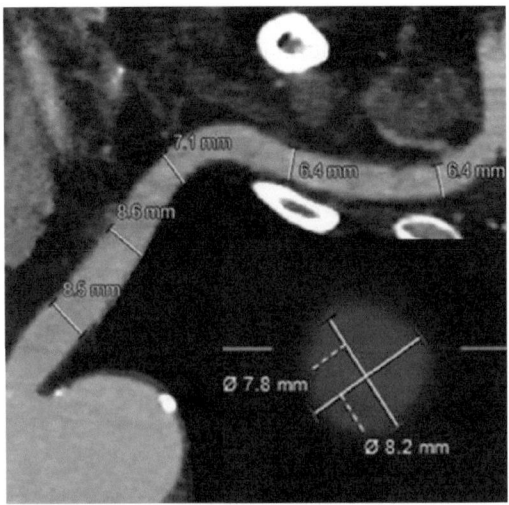

FIGURE 8.1 Trans-subclavian sizing for TAVR access

soften the angle at which the device enters the artery and facilitate access. In percutaneous cases, access should be pre-closed with two Perclose ProGlide™ (Abbott Vascular, Santa Clara, CA) devices. Some have described a through-and-through brachial to femoral safety wire in case stenting is necessary to achieve hemostasis [5]. The subclavian has similar sizing requirements as the femoral which can be determined with 3-D image reconstruction. For example, a minimal arterial diameter of 5.5 mm is required for SAPIEN 3 sizes 20–16 mm or Evolut Pro sizes 23–29. Measuring the size of the axillary, subclavian, and innominate arteries (in right-sided cases) throughout the device course is essential. The course of arterial access should be free of significant calcifications or tortuosity. Examining the *angle of the origin* of the subclavian artery is also necessary [7]. The optimal left subclavian access for TAVR, as in the figure below, is angled slightly toward the left thoracic outlet. A 90° or steeper origin from the aortic arch may be difficult to navigate. The left subclavian generally has better angulation toward the aortic valve for access and deployment and should be preferred to the right subclavian artery. If using the right subclavian artery, a very upright aortic annulus (opposite of horizontal heart) is required. The right subclavian artery may be preferred in cases of myocardial perfusion dependence on a left internal mammary artery bypass graft. If a *mammary graft* is present and the right subclavian is not suitable, a large, >7 mm left subclavian artery allowing perfusion around a large-bore sheath is feasible but should be considered very high risk.

Carotid

Initial reports show transcarotid access to have acceptable outcomes, better than transapical procedures [4, 8]. It is unclear if transcarotid access leads to increased periprocedural stroke. A recent study with 96 patients demonstrates a 6.3% 30-day stroke or TIA rate [9], while other series show 0–3% [10]. The right carotid has a less angled course to the aortic valve, but either side can be used. Exposure is along the medial boarder of the sternocleidomastoid muscle as done for a carotid endarterectomy. Reports have described both clamping of the carotid with cerebral monitoring and shunting of blood from the femoral artery to the distal internal carotid artery. The carotid should be repaired with bovine pericardium to prevent any stenosis following TAVR. This is still a new technique described in few patient numbers.

Data is still emerging regarding the optimal alternative access for TAVR. Reports of successful transcaval aortic access, using a vascular occlusion device to close an iatrogenic aortocaval fistula, have been promising as well [11]. Performing skilled, safe transfemoral as well as alternative access sites will be necessary to perform TAVR.

References

1. Reardon MJ, Van Mieghem NM, Popma JJ, Kleiman NS, Søndergaard L, Mumtaz M, Adams DH, Deeb GM, Maini B, Gada H, Chetcuti S, Gleason T, Heiser J, Lange R, Merhi W, Oh JK, Olsen PS, Piazza N, Williams M, Windecker S, Yakubov

SJ, Grube E, Makkar R, Lee JS, Conte J, Vang E, Nguyen H, Chang Y, Mugglin AS, Serruys PW, Kappetein AP, Investigators SURTAVI. Surgical or transcatheter aortic-valve replacement in intermediate-risk patients. N Engl J Med. 2017;376(14):1321–31.

2. Thourani VH, Kodali S, Makkar RR, Herrmann HC, Williams M, Babaliaros V, Smalling R, Lim S, Malaisrie SC, Kapadia S, Szeto WY, Greason KL, Kereiakes D, Ailawadi G, Whisenant BK, Devireddy C, Leipsic J, Hahn RT, Pibarot P, Weissman NJ, Jaber WA, Cohen DJ, Suri R, Tuzcu EM, Svensson LG, Webb JG, Moses JW, Mack MJ, Miller DC, Smith CR, Alu MC, Parvataneni R, D'Agostino RB Jr, Leon MB. Transcatheter aortic valve replacement versus surgical valve replacement in intermediate-risk patients: a propensity score analysis. Lancet. 2016;387(10034):2218–25.

3. Thourani VH, Jensen HA, Babaliaros V, Suri R, Vemulapalli S, Dai D, Brennan JM, Rumsfeld J, Edwards F, Tuzcu EM, Svensson L, Szeto WY, Herrmann H, Kirtane AJ, Kodali S, Cohen DJ, Lerakis S, Devireddy C, Sarin E, Carroll J, Holmes D, Grover FL, Williams M, Maniar H, Shahian D, Mack M. Transapical and transaortic transcatheter aortic valve replacement in the United States. Ann Thorac Surg. 2015;100(5):1718–26.

4. Thourani VH, Li C, Devireddy C, Jensen HA, Kilgo P, Leshnower BG, Mavromatis K, Sarin EL, Nguyen TC, Kanitkar M, Guyton RA, Block PC, Maas AL, Simone A, Keegan P, Merlino J, Stewart JP, Lerakis S, Babaliaros V. High-risk patients with inoperative aortic stenosis: use of transapical, transaortic, and transcarotid techniques. Ann Thorac Surg. 2015;99(3):817–23; discussion 823-5.

5. Schäfer U, Deuschl F, Schofer N, Frerker C, Schmidt T, Kuck KH, Kreidel F, Schirmer J, Mizote I, Reichenspurner H, Blankenberg S, Treede H, Conradi L. Safety and efficacy of the percutaneous transaxillary access for transcatheter aortic valve implantation using various transcatheter heart valves in 100 consecutive patients. Int J Cardiol. 2017;232:247–54.

6. Petronio AS, De Carlo M, Bedogni F, Maisano F, Ettori F, Klugmann S, Poli A, Marzocchi A, Santoro G, Napodano M, Ussia GP, Giannini C, Brambilla N, Colombo A. 2-year results of CoreValve implantation through the subclavian access: a propensity-matched comparison with the femoral access. J Am Coll Cardiol. 2012;60(6):502–7.

7. Schofer N, Deuschl F, Conradi L, Lubos E, Schirmer J, Reichenspurner H, Blankenberg S, Treede H, Schäfer U. Preferential short cut or alternative route: the transaxillary

access for transcatheter aortic valve implantation. J Thorac Dis. 2015;7(9):1543–7.

8. Kirker EB1, Hodson RW1, Spinelli KJ2, Korngold EC. The carotid artery as a preferred alternative access route for transcatheter aortic valve replacement. Ann Thorac Surg. 2017;104(2):621–9.

9. Mylotte D, Sudre A, Teiger E, Obadia JF, Lee M, Spence M, Khamis H, Al Nooryani A, Delhaye C, Amr G, Koussa M, Debry N, Piazza N, Modine T. Transcarotid transcatheter aortic valve replacement: feasibility and safety. JACC Cardiovasc Interv. 2016;9(5):472–80.

10. Stonier T, Harrison M, Choong AM. A systematic review of transcatheter aortic valve implantation via carotid artery access. Int J Cardiol. 2016;219:41–55.

11. Greenbaum AB, Babaliaros VC, Chen MY, Stine AM, Rogers T, O'Neill WW, Paone G, Thourani VH, Muhammad KI, Leonardi RA, Ramee S, Troendle JF, Lederman RJ. Transcaval access and closure for transcatheter aortic valve replacement: a prospective investigation. J Am Coll Cardiol. 2017;69(5):511–21.

Chapter 9
Wires, Catheters, and Cath Lab Rules

Tables 9.1 and 9.2 provide a quick reference for some of the tools used in TAVR procedures. Getting in the lab and understanding when to use what is the best way to learn. While these capture the most basic interventional cardiology tools, the variety of wire and catheters is endless. Wires come in a variety of sizes (0.018″, 0.025″, 0.032″, 0.035″) and lengths (40, 150, 180, 260, 300 cm). For the vast majority of interventions, you will use an *0.035″* wire and 150 or 260 length. A variety of stiff wires are available for TAVR. While we use the double-curved Lunderquist, finding one that you like and using it repeatedly is critical. Understanding the feel, shape, and pushability of your stiff wire is much more important than which one you use. Likewise, there are catheters in nearly every shape possible available to interventionalists. TAVR procedures utilize mostly 5 and *6 Fr.* catheters. Table 9.2 below highlights those most frequently used by cardiologists. Experience in interventional radiology or vascular surgery will increase your armamentarium and knowledge of catheters. Ultimately, skilled use of a few catheters to perform any interventional maneuver will be much more valuable than knowledge of every catheter out there.

© Springer International Publishing AG, part of Springer Nature 2018
A. C. Watkins et al., *Transcatheter Aortic Valve Replacement*, https://doi.org/10.1007/978-3-319-93396-2_9

TABLE 9.1 Wires used in TAVR

		Properties	Common uses
Micropuncture		Softest, fine	Arterial access Arterial pressure monitoring
Glidewire		Softest, hydrophilic	Navigating atherosclerosis Crossing AV

J wire

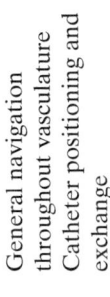

Soft, atraumatic

General navigation throughout vasculature
Catheter positioning and exchange

Amplatz
Extra stiff

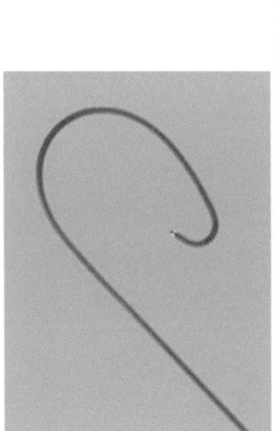

Stiffer than J wire
Softer than super stiff
Soft tip
J, straight or curved

Support for delivery system
Support for TAVR device across AV

(continued)

TABLE 9.1 (continued)

		Properties	Common uses
Amplatz Super stiff		Stiffer than ExtraStiff Softer than Lunderquist Soft tip J straight or curved	Support for delivery system Support for TAVR device across AV
Lunderquist		Stiffest of all wires Straight, curved, or double curved	Support for delivery system Support for TAVR device across AV

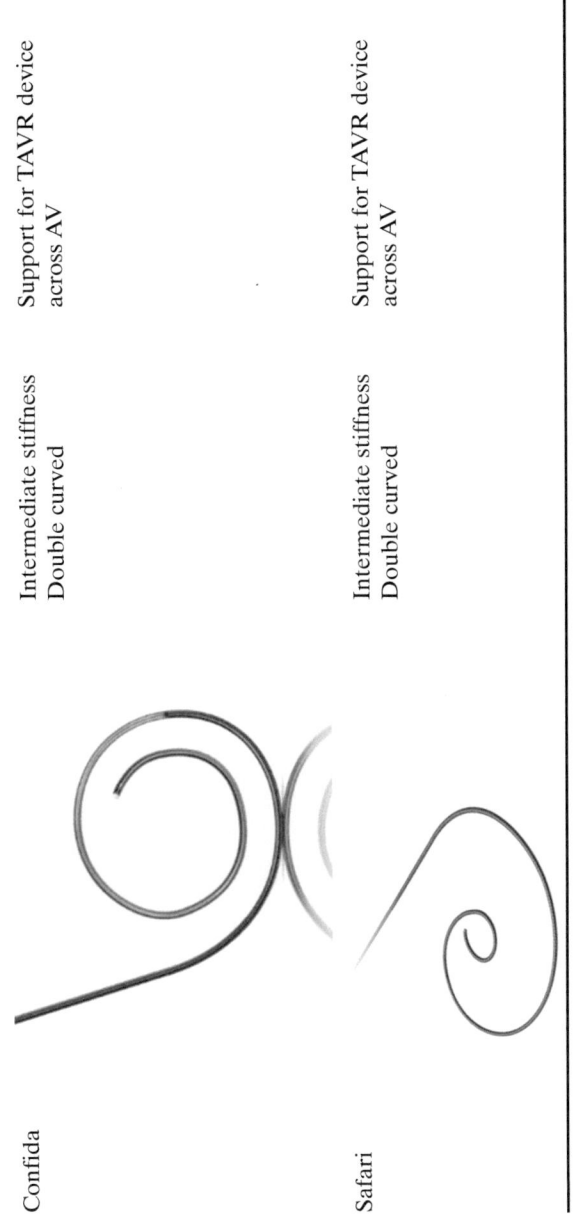

Confida

Intermediate stiffness
Double curved

Support for TAVR device
across AV

Safari

Intermediate stiffness
Double curved

Support for TAVR device
across AV

Table 9.2 Catheters used in TAVR

		Properties	Common uses
Pigtail		Multiple side holes Straight or angled	Aortogram Ventriculogram
Amplatz left			LMCA angiogram Crossing the AV

TABLE 9.2 (continued)

	Properties	Common uses
Judkins right		RMCA angiogram
Judkins left		LMCA angiogram
Omni flush	Multiple side holes 180° angle	Contralateral iliofemoral access/angiogram

Common Cath Lab Rules for CT Surgeons

1. Before initiating fluoroscopy, verify everyone in the room has lead on. Of the course of a career, radiation exposure is a significant occupational hazard. Taking all precautions, using shielding as much as possible and limiting radiation dose will protect your patient, staff, and yourself.
2. Wipe all wires being used with a wet gauze between each catheter passing or any time you think of it.
3. Aspirate and flush each newly introduced catheter with heparinized saline. Air within the catheter can embolize if not removed properly.
4. Use fluoroscopy anytime you are advancing a wire or catheter. There is no reason to find out if your wire is stuck in/perforated a hepatic vein or that your catheter is hubbed in the left main coronary artery after the complication has happened.
5. Hold pressure on the femoral vessels at the end of the case. Despite the assistance of vascular closure devices, manual pressure is always prudent. As in open surgery, minor bleeding often resolves with holding pressure.
6. *Heparin dosing* for endovascular procedures and TAVR: 100 U/Kg. Goal ACT = 300.
7. *Contrast use:* Power injectors are used to overcome resistance in long catheters and deliver contrast faster than one could by hand, allowing a sufficient volume of contrast to produce clear angiography. They are often connected to the back of catheters with a manifold and flush port and must be de-aired every time they are hooked up. Some inject when a plunger or botton is pushed, and others are programmed to inject when cine fluoroscopy starts. Power injectors are programmed to deliver a rate of contrast (mL/second) for a specified volume (mL).

Example: "10 for 20." The patient will receive 10 mL/s of contrast until 20 mL is delivered, which will be 2 s.

Chapter 10
Procedural Considerations and Technical Details

Roles of Participants

TAVR procedures are generally done with both interventional cardiology and cardiac surgery, often two attendings and two fellows scrubbed. This collaboration should be embraced as it offers greater knowledge and experience both in routine TAVR deployment and those complicated by cardiac arrest or vascular injury. The role of the cardiac surgeon may vary among institutions. Again, we recommend involving yourself with all aspects of the TAVR procedure, not just emergencies, in order to practice this new, critical aspect to aortic valve surgery.

Femoral Vessel Access

Fluoroscopy is the modality of choice for directed femoral artery access in interventional cardiology. Ultrasound can be a helpful addition and should be readily available.

Palpate the pulse along the inguinal ligament. It will lie at the medial 1/3 between the anterior superior iliac spine of the pelvis and the pubic symphysis. Place a straight clamp in the direction of the artery at the location of the pulse. Confirm on fluoroscopy that the location of the pulse/clamp lies within

© Springer International Publishing AG, part of Springer Nature 2018
A. C. Watkins et al., *Transcatheter Aortic Valve Replacement*,
https://doi.org/10.1007/978-3-319-93396-2_10

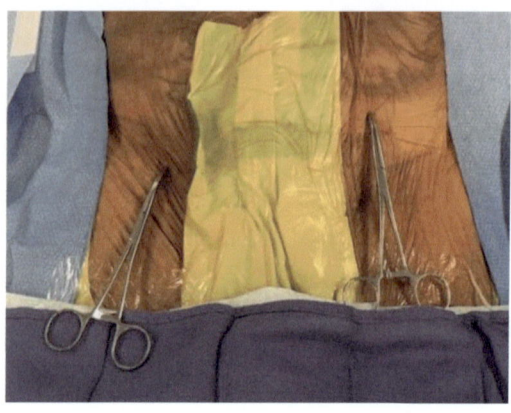

FIGURE 10.1 Setup for fluoroscopy-guided arterial access

the femoral head. Adjust your intended arterial stick location cranial or caudal if not over the femoral head. A higher or lower stick in relation to the femoral head may be preferred based on the quality and location of the common femoral artery as seen on CT scan (Fig. 10.1).

1. Access femoral artery with micropuncture needle aiming for the center of the vessel as to not skive the side of the vessel. With return of bright red blood, gently advance the thin micropuncture wire while visualizing under fluoroscopy. If there is resistance to threading the wire, try slightly lowering the angle of needle, rotating bevel of needle in a different direction, or readvancing the wire with a gentle twist in either direction.
2. Exchange the needle for the 5 Fr micropuncture catheter. Advance a write to verify arterial, not venous access.
3. At this point, the micropuncture sheath is changed out to a 6 Fr. sheath.
4. For any TAVR procedure, both femoral arteries will need to be accessed. One will be dilated to the size of the delivery system, 14 Fr or greater. The other artery will be accessed with a 6 Fr sheath to allow a diagnostic pigtail catheter to

parallel the device providing angiograms of root and positioning of AV during TAVR deployment.
5. Venous access should be obtained with a 6 Fr sheath in either the non-device side of the femoral vein or the right internal jugular vein. This will be for temporary pacemaker access.

Femoral Artery Closure Devices

There are a variety of arterial closure devices available, including Angio-Seal (St Jude, St Paul, MN), Mynx (Cardinal Health, Dublin, OH), Prostar XL and Perclose ProGlide (both by Abbott Vascular, Santa Clara, CA) (Fig. 10.2), and the new MANTA device (Essential Medical, Exton, PN). Mechanisms of closure devices include filling arteriotomy with sealant plug or gel or actively closing hole with a clip or sutures. You must ensure your closure device can adequately close the arteriotomy, which currently for TAVR is at mini-

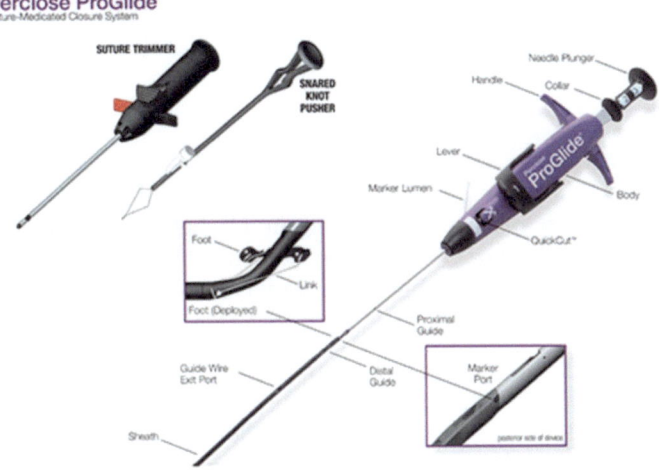

FIGURE 10.2 Perclose ProGlide® closure device by Abbott Vascular (Santa Clara, CA). (Used with permission from Abbott)

mum 18 Fr. This size arteriotomy generally requires a suture closure device. The most commonly used suture device approved for arteriotomy of this size is the Perclose ProGlide system (5–21 Fr). This device deploys a preformed knot of monofilament suture across the hole in the artery.

After arterial access is gained and a 6 Fr sheath is in place, a sheath wire should be placed in the sheath. On withdrawal of the 6 Fr sheath, a skin incision should be placed at the site of the skin, and the skin spread with a small clamp to ensure that there is enough room for the closure devices to deploy without catching skin or subcutaneous tissue. Placing two sutures at 10 and 2 o'clock on the arteriotomy, *prior* to dilation of the arteriotomy for large-bore sheath or device insertion, is a common method. Closure of an arteriotomy over 14 Fr requires two sutures be placed and some choose to use three. Familiarize yourself with the use of this device to ensure successful hemostasis following large-bore dilation of the femoral artery. Some of the vascular closure devices treating smaller arteriotomies can be used for the non-device side. When securing your closure device at the end of the case, *never lose wire access* until you are confident you have achieved hemostasis. This allows endovascular hemostasis and management of your arteriotomy.

Pacing

Ventricular pacing is required in all balloon-expandable TAVR procedures in order to decrease the motion of the aortic valve and annulus during deployment and is often used with the self-expanding TAVR device (Fig. 10.3).

1. With the balloon deflated, a transvenous, endocardial pacemaker is inserted into the venous sheath. Once outside the sheath in the femoral vein, the balloon is inflated and the catheter is floated under fluoroscopy up to the right atrium.
2. Point the catheter toward the tricuspid valve with a clockwise turn and gentle forward advancement. Advance the pacemaker across the valve. Tricuspid regurgitation can

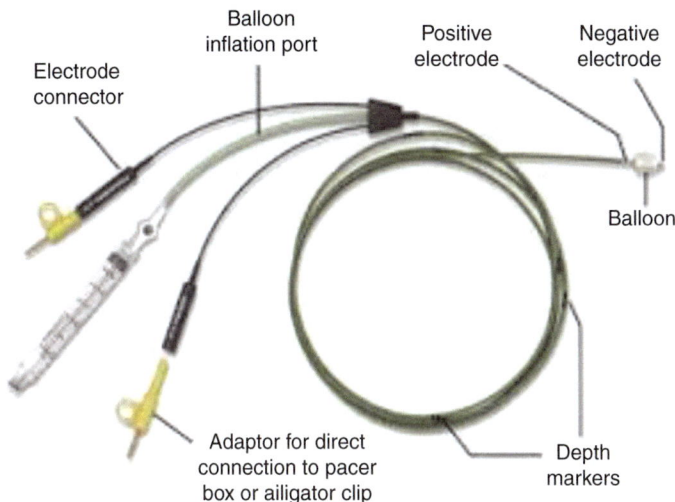

FIGURE 10.3 Transvenous pacemaker

make placing the pacemaker difficult and will require a firmer push. If the approach to the tricuspid valve is angulated, try removing the pacemaker and manually curving the distal end in a round, soft shape to facilitate turning toward the valve.

3. The catheter can be advanced a few more centimeters in the right ventricle aiming toward the apex. Stop advancing the catheter if you feel any resistance or are pointed toward left-sided structures.

4. Deflate the balloon once in the ventricle; never withdraw the pacemaker with the balloon inflated as you could damage the tricuspid valve.

Pigtail Placement and Heparinization

1. After access is obtained and before instrumenting the aortic arch, give 100 U/kg *heparin*. Check ACT; the goal is 250–300 s.

2. A 6 Fr pigtail catheter should be advanced through the nondelivery side femoral artery over a 0.035″ J wire.
3. Once in the ascending aorta, the wire can be withdrawn allowing the pigtail to coil into position.
4. Advance the pigtail to the non-coronary or right sinus of Valsalva. SAPIEN 3 valves are generally deployed with the pigtail in the right sinus, while Evolut Pro valves are deployed with the pigtail in the non-coronary sinus. It usually goes preferentially to the non-coronary sinus, but the outside end of the catheter can be turned in either direction to aid landing in the correct sinus.

Crossing the Aortic Valve

1. At this point, any further maneuvers to *confirm the delivery angle* can be done, including an aortic root *angiogram* and additional pigtail placement in the right coronary sinus [1] (Fig. 10.4). LAO 30° CRA 0° often is a good place to start.
2. Depending on your valve choice, this may be done before or after placement of the femoral sheath or delivery sys-

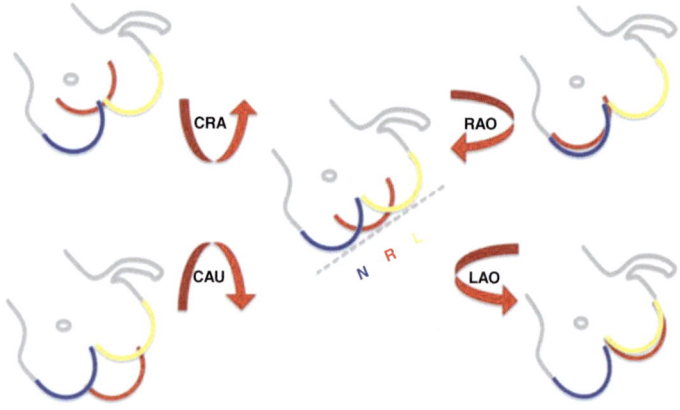

FIGURE 10.4 Gantry maneuvers to find optimal deployment angle. (Reprinted from Kasel et al. [1], with permission from Elsevier)

tem. The SAPIEN 3 delivery system is usually introduced before crossing the valve, while the Evolut Pro is after.

3. Advance a 6 Fr *AL-1* catheter over a J wire to the aortic root using the delivery access.

4. Position your fluoroscopy at the predetermined *deployment angle*.

5. Exchange the J wire for a *straight 0.035" Glidewire*. Crossing of the aortic valve should be done with a straight wire.

6. Visualize the leaflets of the valve opening and closing on fluoroscopy. Point the AL-1 at the center of the valve, and softly advance the Glidewire toward the ventricle.

7. Repeat this until the wire crosses into the ventricle. When the wire hits the valve leaflets and sinuses, stop, retract the wire, and rotate the catheter slightly to try again. Do not push the wire forcefully against valve or coil the wire in the sinuses.

8. If your catheter approach doesn't work, rotate the catheter clockwise or counterclockwise, moving the distal end of the catheter across the aortic root, and try again. If crossing the valve is still difficult, you can exchange the AL-1 for a JR4 or AL-2 catheter to change the angle at which you approach the valve.

9. Once the wire is across, gently advance the *catheter into the mid-ventricle*. Aspirate the catheter. If blood doesn't withdraw, the end of your catheter is against the wall of the ventricle. Rotate the catheter away until you can withdraw blood.

10. Now with your pigtail in the aortic root and catheter in the ventricle, acquire baseline hemodynamic measurements. This will be helpful to compare to post-TVAR *hemodynamics*.

11. Exchange the straight Glidewire for the preferred delivery wire (e.g., double-curve Lunderquist). The delivery wire should be further pre-curled prior to entry into the catheter. In patients with a very small ventricle, a softer wire might be preferred to avoid perforation. Gently advance wire into apex with a round, atraumatic shape (Fig. 10.5).

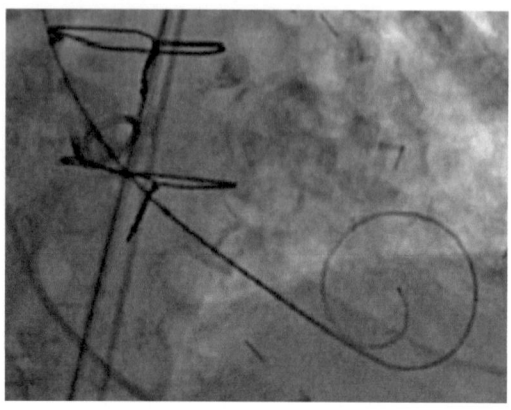

FIGURE 10.5 Ideal position of stiff left ventricular wire for TAVR. (Used with permission from Medtronic)

Pre-TAVR Balloon Aortic Valvuloplasty

A primary goal in a successful TAVR deployment is maintaining hemodynamic stability. If the AV is stenotic such that placement of the device will cause hemodynamic collapse (or would make it difficult for the valve to cross), pre-TAVR balloon valvuloplasty (BAV) should be performed. An important consideration is that a BAV can cause hemodynamically significant aortic insufficiency. Prior to performing a BAV, *have the TAVR system preprepared.* There are many valvuloplasty balloons available. Commonly used balloon are the True Balloon (Bard Medical, Covington, GA) and the Z-MED balloon (B. Braun Medical, Bethlehem, PA). The True balloon is non-compliant while the Z-MED is semi-compliant (Fig. 10.6).

1. Ensure the pigtail catheter is in the non-coronary sinus.
2. Select a balloon *less than* or equal to the smallest diameter of your aortic annulus. With significant annular or LVOT calcium, choose a smaller balloon to prevent annular rupture. Especially with a non-compliant True balloon, you

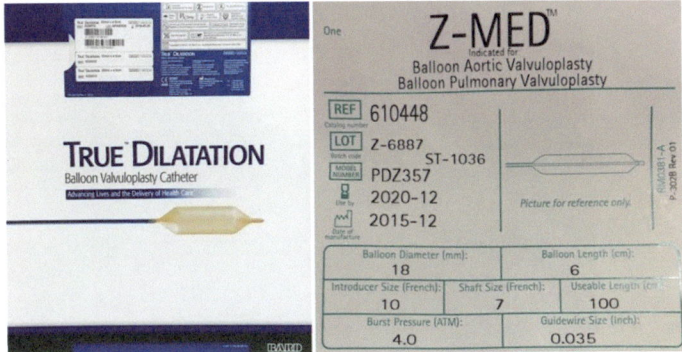

FIGURE 10.6 Balloons used in pre-TAVR balloon aortic valvuloplasty

should pick a size at least 2 mm smaller than your annulus. It is always prudent to choose a smaller balloon, as you are only trying to open the valve enough to safely fit the device through it.

3. Advance the balloon over the stiff wire into the left ventricle, positioned evenly across the aortic valve.
4. Load the inflation syringe of the balloon with a 10% contrast/heparinized saline mix.
5. One operator maintains the position of the balloon, while another will inflate the balloon.
6. Rapid pace at a rate limiting cardiac output, generally 160–220 beats/min.
7. Inflate the balloon, stopping when you meet resistance. Apply gentle forward pressure on the balloon catheter as the balloon goes up as cardiac output will tend to push the balloon out.

SAPIEN 3 Delivery System

1. This is done *prior to crossing the valve*, or any BAV.
2. Advance an AL-1 over a J wire to the ascending aorta.
3. Exchange the J wire for a stiff wire; we use a double-curved *Lunderquist*.

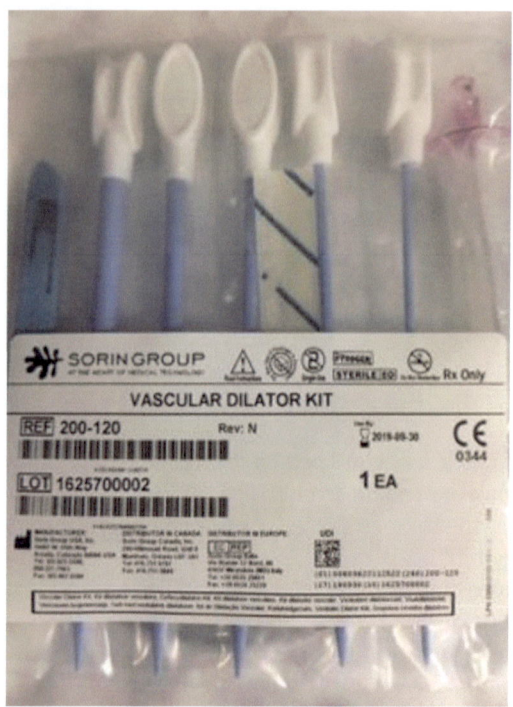

FIGURE 10.7 Sorin Dilator Kit

4. Remove the AL-1 and serially dilate the femoral arteriotomy to a 12 Fr size. We like the *Sorin Vascular Dilator Kit* (LivaNova, London, UK) (Fig. 10.7):

5. Slowly advance the Edwards eSheath (14 Fr expands to 18 Fr) while watching the femorals, iliacs, and aorta *under fluoroscopy*. The inner dilator (white) does not fix to the sheath (blue) requiring one hand on the back of the catheter to maintain the dilator position. Stop advancing if you see any bending or kinking of the wire or meet any resistance. Do not withdraw the catheter unless you plan in abandoning a femoral approach; multiple passes will increase the risk of vascular complication.

6. When the sheath is in the abdominal aorta, remove the inner dilator. Secure to the skin.

Evolut Pro Delivery System

There are two ways to deliver the Evolut R to the aorta: through an additional sheath or using the in-line sheath ("bareback"). If the size of the femoral and iliac arteries allows an 18 Fr sheath and the team is more comfortable with hemostasis provided by a sheath, there are a few very similar choices. We have had success with the Cook's Check-Flo® Sheath. However, because the in-line sheath of the Evolut Pro allows a low risk of vascular complication, we prefer to use only the in-line sheath unless substantial tortuosity requires the use of a sheath.

1. The Evolut Pro is introduced *after crossing the AV* with the stiff wire, and after any BAV.
2. *Zoom out* the magnification of the fluoroscopy ("mag out") to visualize both the curved wire in the left ventricle and the iliacs.
3. *Inspect the valve* under fluoroscopy while rotating 360° to ensure (Fig. 10.8):

   (a) The capsule is not overdriven. There should be a small gap.
   (b) The paddles are squarely in the sockets and are 180° apart.
   (c) All markers in the stent frame are straight.

   If the paddles are malaligned, there may be instability when the device is released or inability to recapture the valve.

4. Dilate the femoral arteriotomy to a 16 Fr size with the Sorin dilators.

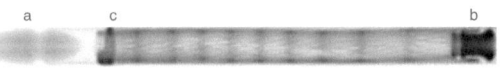

Figure 10.8 Fluoroscopic markers of Evolut valve. (**a**) Capsule. (**b**) Paddles. (**c**) Hat marker and stent frames. (Used with permission from Medtronic)

5. Slowly advance the valve and in-line sheath into the abdominal aorta while watching under fluoroscopy. Stop advancing if you see any bending or kinking of the wire or meet any resistance.

Second Time-Out

At our institution, we employ a second opportunity, immediately before the valve is positioned, to ensure that all participants are prepared and that all necessary equipment is readily available. Below is our checklist (Fig. 10.9):

SURGICAL TIME OUT

☐ PATIENT IDENTIFIERS: NAME & DOB

☐ PROCEDURE IDENTIFIED: VALVE SIZE/APPROACH

☐ PATIENT ALLERGIES DISCUSSED

BEFORE VALVE IS INTRODUCED

☐ CONFIRM ANTIBIOTIC GIVEN

☐ 4 UNITS OF BLOOD IN ROOM?

☐ BYPASS CANNULA SIZES AVAILABLE?

☐ ACCESS SITE IDENTIFIED? WHO WILL HAND OFF?

☐ CORONARY EQUIPMENT IDENTIFIED? HANDING OFF?

☐ VALVULOPLASTY BALLOON LENGTH & SIZE?_____ (not usually done for Medtronic)

☐ WHO'S PACING? WHO'S GIVING THE DIRECTIONS?

☐ DEFIBRILLATOR PAD PLACED AXILLARY/TURNED ON AND HOOKED UP? WHO IS DEFIBRILLATING?

☐ PERFUSIONIST AVAILABLE?

☐ ECHOCARDIOGRAPHER IN ROOM?

☐ PROCEDURAL CONSIDERATIONS TO BE AWARE OF: ANY ATRIAL APPENDAGE thrombus? COPD? RENAL FCT? GRAFT STATUS? PACEMAKER?

☐ ECHO FINDINGS: ANNULUS_____ & VALVE SIZE

☐ CONFIRM THAT ORIENTATION HAS BEEN CHECKED BY PHYSICIAN (Edwards) OR THAT VALVE HAS BEEN CHECKED UNDER FLUORO (Medtronic Evolut)

☐ STERNAL SAW HOOKED UP AND TESTED?

☐ PERICARDIOCENTESIS KIT IN ROOM? (for TF cases ONLY)

☐ ARE THE AORTIC, ILIAC & FEMORAL BALLOONS & STENTS PULLED? WHO'S RESPONSIBLE FOR HANDING OFF? (for TF cases ONLY)

FIGURE 10.9 Second time-out checklist

SAPIEN 3 Deployment

As the most important and often unstable moment of the procedure, clear directions by team leader as to sequence of events during deployment are critical. With extended time in the valve crimper or loaded in the Commander delivery system, there is increased risk of leaflet damage. Prepare the valve at this point, immediately prior to use [2].

1. Advance the valve to the descending thoracic aorta while watching on fluoroscopy. This will require a significant push while the valve is within and expanding the eSheath. The Edwards logo should point up to the ceiling.
2. Unlock the locking mechanism on the delivery advance. Withdraw the balloon into the valve. A *white mark* will be exposed on the balloon catheter. Lock the delivery system.
3. Using the *fine-tuning knob*, position the balloon in the center of the valve. Fluoroscopic markers at the ends and center of the balloon will serve as a guide.
4. Lock and unlock the delivery system to release any *stored tension* in the system. Stored tension can lead to instability in crossing the valve or deploying the device.
5. Advance the transcatheter valve over the aortic arch and through the aortic valve. If length of the device is inadequate, there is a peel-away loader that can be removed. One operator should steadily advance the valve while another turns the *flex knob* on the delivery system, conforming the shape of the arch and minimizing trauma. This may be facilitated by a gentle outward pull on the wire. If you encounter resistance at the aortic valve annulus or any point or see any abnormal bending of the nose cone, stop. You may get across by readjusting the flex on the device and trying again with a constant firm pressure forward. You may need to do a balloon valvuloplasty if unable to safely get the transcatheter valve positioned.

6. Adjust the fluoroscopy projection to your predetermined deployment angle and shoot an *angiogram* of the aortic root if necessary to confirm coplanar view.
7. Unlock the delivery system and withdraw the flexible catheter back away from the balloon so it doesn't interfere with deployment. Relock the delivery system.
8. Release some of the flex to position the valve in the center of the annulus, and *position the valve 3–5 mm below the annulus.* When deployed, ideally 80–90% of the valve will be on the aortic side of the annulus and *10–20% ventricular.* Keep in mind the valve will *foreshorten from the bottom* up. Prior to deployment, while the center marker is near the annulus, the ventricular edge of the valve will move closer to the annulus. At our institution, we put the center marker just above the annulus with the goal of 3–5 mm of stent below the annulus after deployment (Fig. 10.10).
9. With the device across the valve but not deployed, hemodynamics may be jeopardized, making clear directions and expeditious deployment necessary. At any point if

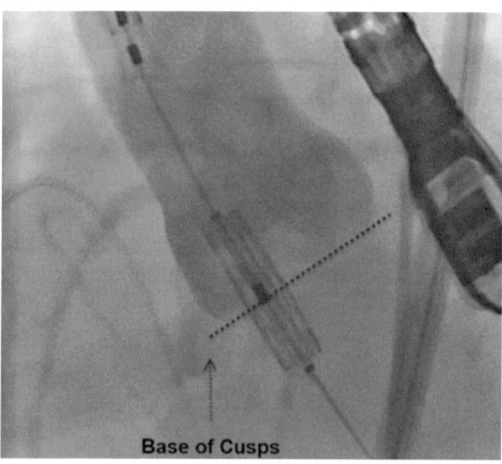

FIGURE 10.10 Positioning of SAPIEN 3 for deployment. (Used with permission from Edwards Lifesciences)

hemodynamic are unacceptable or the team is not ready to deploy, the valve should simply be withdrawn back into the ascending aorta and the patient's vital signs allowed to recover. Anesthesia can also support hemodynamics with premedication with vasoconstrictors.

10. Deployment:

   (a) *Rapid pacing:* Hold ventilation.
   (b) Initiate pacing at *160–220 beat/second.*
   (c) *Angiogram* through pigtail using power injector. 35 cc/second for a total of 10–15 cc is generally adequate.
   (d) *Positioner:* Maintain the device at the intended depth, 3–5 mm, with the center marker slightly above the annulus. This is done with both gentle pressure on the device in the intended direction and slight movement of the wire in the opposite direction. When the valve is crimped in the delivery system, its length is stretch out. When deployed, it foreshortens to a shorter height. The valve will usually tend to foreshorten in the direction of the aorta. Make sure you are using the sinus nadirs as your visual marker and not a piece of calcium that could move during deployment. Radiographic markers in the center of the SAPIEN 3 valve will serve as you visual valve markers.
   (e) *Deployer:* Release the lock on the insufflator. The nominal inflation volume for the balloon is located on the green, end part of the delivery system. Inflate balloon slowly initially allowing the positioner to react to any movement of the device. Once the valve appears to have adhered to the annulus, a more forceful inflation fully expands the valve. Hold the inflation for 3–4 s, and then quickly deflate the balloon.
   (f) *Pigtail:* Either the positioner or a third operator withdraws the pigtail as the valve expands [4]. The valve pictured below is positioned at roughly 10 mm on the left sinus and 12 mm on the non-coronary sinus. Its position is 70% aortic and 30% ventricular (Fig. 10.11).

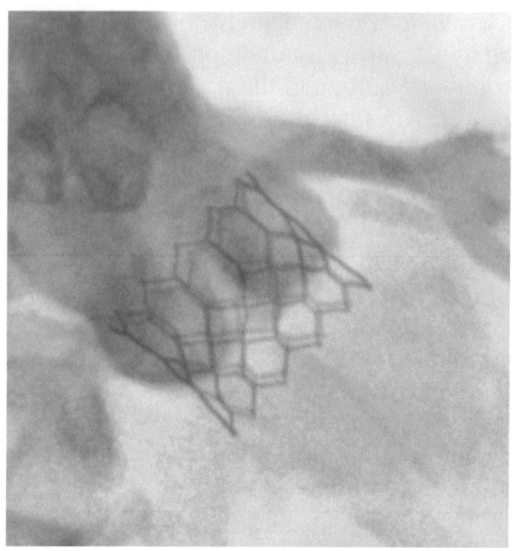

FIGURE 10.11 SAPIEN 3 TAVR deployed "30% ventricular and 70% aortic." (Used with permission from Edwards Lifesciences)

11. Withdraw the delivery system back into the descending aorta. Assess the valve for position and perivalvular leak, using echocardiogram, angiogram, and hemodynamics. If satisfactory, withdraw the delivery system back into sheath and remove. Put the dilator back in the sheath.
12. Remove the sheath and close the arteriotomy with the Perclose sutures. Slowly coming down on the Perclose sutures over the taper of the dilator as it is slowly removed can help in allowing the sutures to capture.
13. Access EKG and remove pacemaker if no changes. If any conduction changes, leave pacemaker in for use during recovery.

With either valve type, positioning the valve too ventricular will increase the risk of AV conduction defects and mitral valve dysfunction. A position too aortic will increase the risk of coronary obstruction or device embolization. Positioning either valve is a dynamic process, requiring constant feedback

to any motion of the valve and constant communication with
the operator deploying the valve.

Evolut Pro Deployment

1. Advance the valve over the aortic arch and through the
   aortic valve. There is no flex feature. This should be done in
   one smooth motion and can be facilitated by mild outward
   tension on the stiff wire. If you encounter resistance at the
   aortic valve annulus or any point or see any abnormal
   bending of the nose cone, stop. You may get across by readjusting and rotating the device and trying again with a constant firm pressure forward, or you may need to do a
   balloon valvuloplasty [3].
2. With the fluoroscopy projection to your predetermined
   deployment angle, shoot an *angiogram* of the aortic root.
3. Once across the valve, *position the valve 3 mm below the
   annulus*. Medtronic recommends an implantation depth of
   3–5 mm. In our experience, a depth of 1–3 mm gives good
   results and minimizes conduction defects. The first half-cell
   in the stent frame on the ventricular side of the Evolut Pro
   is *6 mm*. The first whole cell on the ventricular side is
   10 mm. Use these dimensions to guide you.
4. Deployment:

   (a) *Rapid pacing*: The Evolut Pro deployment is more
       deliberate than the SAPIEN 3, due to the self-
       expanding nature of the valve. Pacing can be done at a
       slower rate or for only the first 2/3 of deployment.
   (b) *Angiogram* through pigtail using power injector. 35 cc/
       second with 10–15 cc is generally adequate.
   (c) *Positioner*: Maintain the device at the intended depth,
       approximately 3 mm. This is done with both gentle
       pressure on the device in the intended direction and
       slight movement of the wire in the opposite direction.
       Initially, the device will most commonly try to dive
       ventricular and the positioner must respond. It is
       important that the valve slowly, stably adheres to the

outer curve of the aorta. Once adherent to the outer curve, the device commonly will try to dive in the ventricular direction. Constant, subtle, aortic pulling while the some places forward pressure on the stiff wire allows the stent frame to engage the outer curve of the aorta without losing positon at the annulus. Again, depending on the energy stored in the system, this directionality may change. Maintaining position until the valve is fully released is imperative as paddles are released and position can change even at this last step.

(d) *Deployer*: The valve is deployed by turning the large blue deployment knob in the direction of the arrows. The first 1/3 of the valve deployment should be done very *slowly* as the valve adheres in the correct position. As the valve is uncovered, cardiac output will be obstructed between 1/3 and 2/3 of deployment. Blood pressure will drop and the valve should be *rapidly* deployed between these two points. *Stop* deployment when the capsule is just below the paddles (a marker line is present). An uncovered portion of the stent frame is exposed and the hemodynamics will recover (Fig. 10.12).

(e) At this point, *asses the position* of the valve and evaluate any perivalvular leak (Fig. 10.13). The excessively ventricular valve position shown below was causing new mitral regurgitation as well as perivalvular AI. The valve was recaptured and repositioned more toward the aorta.

(f) At this point, it is also helpful to *release tension* in the system by gently pulling back on the wire. If the valve is satisfactory, very slowly deploy the remaining valve. The two paddles will be the last parts to release. If the position is not optimal or there is a significant perivalvular leak, the valve can be *recaptured* by quickly rotating the deployment knob in the opposite direction. The Evolut Pro valve can be recaptured several times. If recapturing repeatedly, an unusual occurrence, securing a new valve is preferred. Additionally, it is recom-

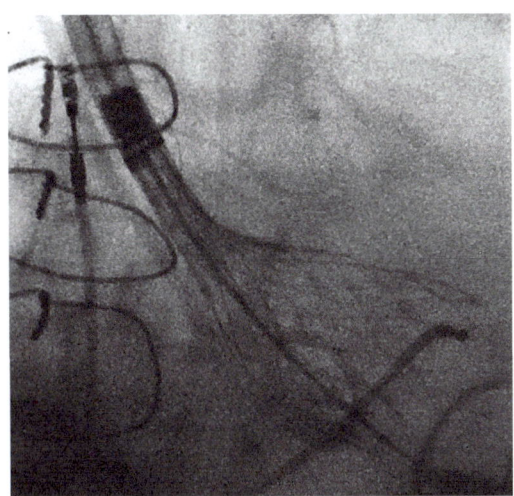

FIGURE 10.12 Evolut R TAVR deployed to the final point of being able to be recaptured

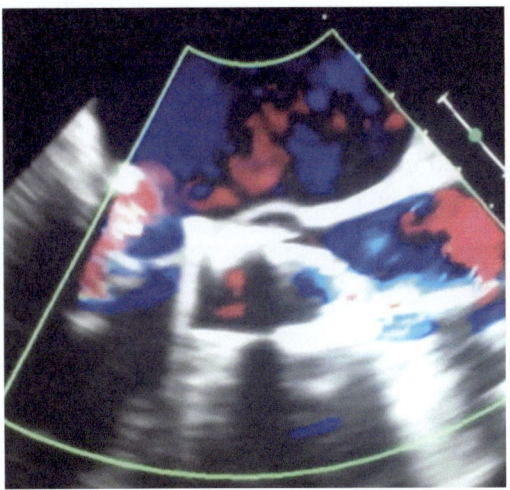

FIGURE 10.13 Echocardiographic evaluation of partially deployed Evolut R TAVR demonstrating paravalvular leak and mitral leaflet interference

mended not to exceed over 15 min between recapture and redeployment to avoid stress on the leaflets.

(g) *Pigtail*: Either the positioner or a third operator, withdraws the pigtail as the valve in expands.

5. Withdraw the delivery system back into the descending aorta. At this point, the delivery system must be *recaptured*. Pull back the gray button on the deployment knob, and then in one smooth motion, pull the entire device backward until flush with deployment knob.

6. Reassess the valve with echocardiogram, angiogram, and hemodynamics to ensure no other work needs to be done.

7. Remove device and close arteriotomy with Perclose closure device.

Assessment and Management of Perivalvular Leak

Aortic insufficiency (AI) is determined with echocardiogram (TEE or TTE) (Fig. 10.14), aortic root angiogram, and hemodynamic assessment. As previously described, the significance of a mild perivalvular leak (PVL) is controversial. However, a moderate or greater is consistently associated with increased mortality. On echo, the aortic valve is examined in the basal short and long axis views:

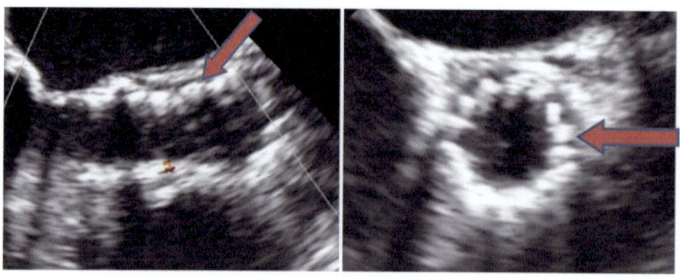

FIGURE 10.14 Echocardiographic evaluation of fully deployed Evolut R TAVR demonstrating no paravalvular leak. (Used with permission from Medtronic)

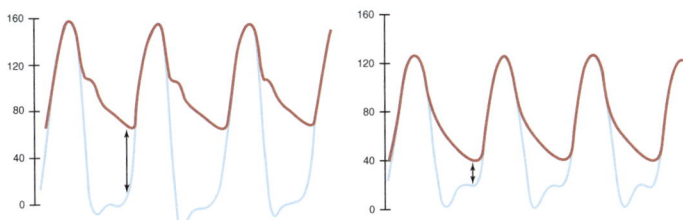

FIGURE 10.15 Red = aortic pressure. Blue = LV pressure. The left shows normal post-TAVR hemodynamics: a low LVEDP (10), a high DBP (80), and an AI Index of 0.58. The right shows significant AI as seen by a depressed DBP (40), elevated LVEDP (20), and an AI Index of 0.17 [5]

Color-flow Doppler will reveal any leaking around the valve. Root angiogram will also confirm your valve position and show the degree and position of any PVL. Hemodynamics taken simultaneously from the aortic root and left ventricle will allow you to assess for significant aortic insufficiency. A low diastolic blood (DBP) pressure and an elevated left ventricular end-diastolic pressure (LVEDP) are signs of aortic insufficiency. More quantitatively, you can calculate an *AI Index*: (DBP – LVEDP)/SBP. A value less than 0.25 is concerning for substantial AI (Fig. 10.15) [5].

The following maneuvers can be used to try to decrease a PVL and should be considered in this order:

1. *Post-TAVR balloon dilatation*: Any mild or greater perivalvular (not central) AI should be treated with balloon dilation. This can be done with either valve type and is similar to a pre-TAVR balloon valvuloplasty. For the SAPIEN 3, it is most conveniently done with the balloon used to deploy the device. For Evolut Pro, any BAV balloon will suffice. If using a non-compliant or True Balloon, undersize balloon 1–2 mm. The degree of any LVOT or aortic calcium will dictate how aggressive to be. Post-TAVR balloon dilation has been shown to decrease moderate or severe perivalvular leak by 75% and has not been shown to have increased neurologic complications [6]. Balloon dilation after TAVR

can also lead to device embolization for an aortically placed valve and to central AI.

2. *Deploy a second valve* in a different position. A deployment that is too aortic in position increases the risk of an AI as well as possible valve embolus with balloon dilation. If a valve is deployed higher than expected and there is moderate or greater perivalvular leak, a second valve may be a safer option than balloon dilation.

3. Successful treatments of perivalvular leaks with a Amplatz ® vascular plug has been reported in high-volume TAVR centers. This may be a helpful option when perivalvular leak is due to eccentric annular calcium or is unresponsive to balloon dilation [7].

References

1. Kasel AM, Cassese S, Leber AW, von Scheidt W, Kastrati A. Fluoroscopy-guided aortic root imaging for TAVR: "follow the right cusp" rule. JACC Cardiovasc Imaging. 2013;6(2):274–5.
2. www.Edwards.com.
3. www.Medtronic.com.
4. Binder RK, Rodés-Cabau J, Wood DA, Mok M, Leipsic J, De Larochellière R, Toggweiler S, Dumont E, Freeman M, Willson AB, Webb JG. Transcatheter aortic valve replacement with the SAPIEN 3: a new balloon-expandable transcatheter heart valve. JACC Cardiovasc Interv. 2013;6(3):293–300.
5. Sinning JM, Hammerstingl C, Vasa-Nicotera M, Adenauer V, Lema Cachiguango SJ, Scheer AC, Hausen S, Sedaghat A, Ghanem A, Müller C, Grube E, Nickenig G, Werner N. Aortic regurgitation index defines severity of peri-prosthetic regurgitation and predicts outcome in patients after transcatheter aortic valve implantation. J Am Coll Cardiol. 2012;59(13):1134–41.
6. Harrison JK, Hughes GC, Reardon MJ, Stoler R, Grayburn P, Hebeler R, Liu D, Chang Y, Popma JJ, CoreValve US. Clinical investigators. Balloon post-dilation following implantation of a self-expanding transcatheter aortic valve bioprosthesis. JACC Cardiovasc Interv. 2017;10(2):168–75.
7. White JM, Khalique OK, Kodali SK. Immediate, same-setting paravalvular leak closure following transcatheter aortic valve replacement. Int J Cardiol. 2015;189:235–7.

Chapter 11
Cardiopulmonary Bypass and Cardiac Surgery in TAVR

Although rare, procedural complication rates are persistently 1–2%. A recent examination of over 15,000 TAVR procedures in Germany reported the rate of severe procedural complications is 5%. This study identified female sex, heart failure, peripheral vascular disease, and heavy calcifications as risk for severe procedural complications [1]. Approximately 50–60% of TAVR patients requiring cardiac surgical intervention survive to discharge [1, 2]. The knowledgeable use of cardiopulmonary bypass or open surgery in TAVR is a requirement of all cardiac surgeons.

The *resuscitation plan* and wishes of the patient should be discussed and clear to all participants prior to any TAVR procedure. There is often very little time for decision-making during following procedural complications, making preoperative communication between the surgeon and patient essential. As TAVR is utilized in younger and lower-risk patients, resuscitation algorithms will be more aggressive. In every elderly, extreme-risk patients, the patient may opt for less aggressive resuscitation measures. Skilled endovascular management of complications is very important in high-risk or inoperative patients. The second-time-out checklist presented previously allows the surgeon and entire team to prepare for the rare event when cardiac surgery or cardiopulmonary bypass is needed. Just as in a routine TAVR procedure, the

© Springer International Publishing AG, part of Springer Nature 2018
A. C. Watkins et al., *Transcatheter Aortic Valve Replacement*,
https://doi.org/10.1007/978-3-319-93396-2_11

roles of all participants in an emergency should be clearly designated prior to starting.

The most common complications requiring resuscitation are cardiac injury causing pericardial bleeding and tamponade or myocardial ischemia resulting from low flow during periods of rapid pacing. The best approach is to meticulously try to prevent catastrophic complications. During an intraprocedural TAVR emergency, there are a few *decisions* to make very quickly:

1. Will this patient *survive*:

   A. CPB?
   B. Sternotomy?
   C. Myocardial arrest and cardiac surgery?
   D. Circulatory arrest?

2. What does the echocardiogram and ECG show?
3. Should we give protamine?
   If intracardiac, annular, or aortic injury is diagnosed or suspected: Yes
   If myocardial ischemia is diagnosed or suspected: No
4. Does the patient need a pericardiocentesis?
   If moderate to large pericardial effusion or any signs of tamponade: Yes
   If reoperative, adherent anatomy or pericardiocentesis cannot be performed safely: No
5. Can we fix this complication endovascularly?
   If vascular injury, appropriate stent available and wire is across injury: Yes
   If coronary ischemia amenable to PCI: Yes
6. Should I cannulate for *ECMO*?
   If cardiac arrest or life-threatening blood pressure or heart rhythm: Yes
   If refused preoperatively: No
7. Should I o*pen the chest*?
   If intracardiac, annular, or aortic injury is diagnosed or suspected: Yes
   If refused preoperatively: No

Annular Rupture

Annular rupture most commonly happens during balloon valvuloplasty, deployment of balloon-expandable valves, or post-TAVR balloon dilation for the management of perivalvular leak. The degree of rupture can vary in severity, from annular hematoma noticed on a post-TAVR CT to complete rupture with immediate tamponade and cardiac arrest. The 1% risk of this dreaded complication is proportional to the extent of annular and *LVOT calcification* and the degree of *oversizing* [3, 4]. Prevention of annular rupture in patients with a heavily calcified annulus or LVOT is best done by using a self-expanding valve and avoiding balloon valvuloplasty. Annular rupture is also more frequent in a small size annulus and severe or asymmetric LV hypertrophy [2]. Stable hematomas in patients at high or prohibitive risk for surgery may be conservatively managed with *heparin reversal*, isolated pericardial drainage, and reevaluation by CT scan. The long-term prognosis for these patients is not known. Severe injury with exposed valve or stent frame may not be survivable. Survivable injuries in low-, intermediate-, or high-risk patients should be treated with standard surgical therapy, including patch reconstruction and valve and aortic root replacement as necessary. Defining the extent of injury through inspection and TEE will dictate repair. Occurring most commonly near LVOT, small hematomas extending into myocardium, but not through epicardium, may be visible on lateral heart or near LAA (Fig. 11.1) [3]. Monitoring for coronary ischemia following annular rupture is important as hematomas may compress the coronary ostia. Depending on the location and extent of a contained rupture, adjacent cardiac structures may be involved. New mitral regurgitation, tricuspid regurgitation, intracardiac shunt, or conduction abnormality should raise concern for annular rupture. Additionally, unnoticed or small hematomas managed medically can develop into LV or aortic pseudoaneurysms over time as pictured below [3].

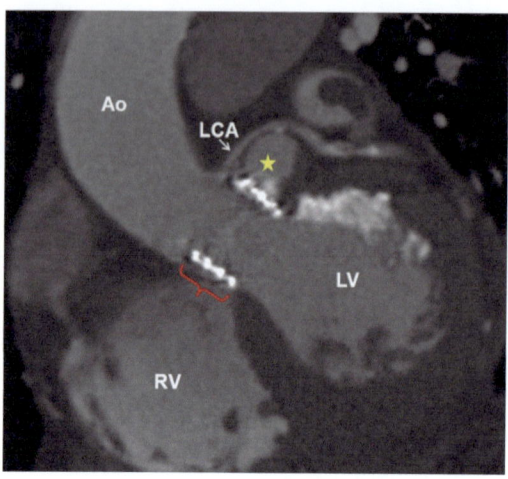

FIGURE 11.1 Contained annular rupture with peri-annular hematoma (Reprinted with permission from Pasic et al. [3])

Ventricular Injury

Left ventricular injuries from wires or devices commonly present with pericardial effusion and tamponade and rarely can be managed without sternotomy. Prevention includes careful, direct visualization of any wires within the left ventricle. The double-curved Lunderquist is the stiffest wire available. In small ventricles, consider using an Amplatz Super Stiff™ (Boston Scientific, Canton, MA) or Confida™ wire (Medtronic, Minneapolis, MN) which are slightly softer. Introducing a generous double bend on the wire prior to use allows multiple loops in the wire with the LV and may prevent wire injury. While there are many features to inspect and monitor while introducing a transcatheter valve, careful monitoring of wire position in the LV is imperative. Upon sternotomy, large injuries will be evident, but small wire injuries can often stop bleeding and be difficult to find. Wire injuries can happen anywhere in LV. Thorough inspection and repair is critical as small wire injuries may reopen with increased blood pressure. Wire injuries can be primarily repaired with full-thickness pledgeted proline. Larger tears from TAVR delivery systems may require cardiopulmonary bypass and myocardial arrest for more extensive repair. Injuries to the right ventricle from the transvenous pacemaker can often be managed conservatively with pericardial drainage, much more frequently than left-sided injuries.

Aortic Injury

Many TAVR patients demonstrate atherosclerosis throughout their vasculature. With multiple passes of wires, catheters, and devices, the aorta is vulnerable to injury anywhere in its course. The risk of aortic dissection is 0.2–0.3% [1, 2]. Outcomes following aortic injury or dissection during TAVR are mostly anecdotal and range from good to death. With injury between the valve and the arch, expeditious *conversion to open* aortic repair is prudent (Table 11.1). Some instances of isolated aortic injury in high-risk patients can be managed with sternotomy, manual pressure, and reversal of heparin, without extensive operation. In low-, intermediate-, and high-risk patients with type A aortic dissections, open repair is necessary. Femoral, axillary, innominate artery and aortic arch cannulations are viable options. Type A *aortic dissection* in inoperable or extreme-risk patients, or patient refusing open surgery, can be

TABLE 11.1 Sternotomy in TAVR

1. Large, enlarging or hemodynamically significant pericardial *effusion*

2. Patient arrests and there any effusion

3. Pericardiocentesis drains continual or substantial amount (>200 mL) of *blood*

4. Patient arrests and the echo nonfunction or inconclusive

5. The patient arrests during rapid pacing or outflow occlusion with no vital signs at 3 min of *CPR*

6. Type A aortic dissection

7. Ascending aorta or arch injury

8. Ongoing myocardial ischemia, need for CABG

medically managed and/or referred for endovascular stenting of the ascending aorta. Likewise, type B aortic dissections or descending or abdominal aortic injuries should be managed according to standard of care. Uncomplicated dissections can be managed medically. Complicated, perforated, or expanding dissections or pseudoaneurysms should be treated with aortic endografting. Abdominal aortic injuries near the visceral vessels may require open surgical control and repair. It is also possible that patients with a small, undiagnosed iatrogenic aortic injury progress to dissection hours or days into the postoperative period due to high blood pressure. Prevention of aortic injuries is best done with careful manipulation of endovascular tools during each step of the TAVR procedure.

Patients with *prior cardiac surgery* have additional considerations when managing iatrogenic injury during TAVR. Firstly, an oscillating saw should be available during TAVR in reoperative patients. If emergent reentry is necessary, it will inevitably take longer than expected. Safe cannulation for *ECMO prior to sternotomy* is recommended. A consideration is that reoperative patients will have pericardial and mediastinal adhesions. Cardiac and aortic injuries are more likely to be contained within scarred anatomy. Conservative management in high-risk, reoperative patients may be more successful than in those without prior surgery. Additionally, reoperative anatomy will vary widely. While review of the preoperative imaging will focus on device compatibility, as the surgeon on the team, working knowledge of reentry anatomy is your responsibility. Patients with prohibitive reoperative anatomy, such as bypass grafts or aorta adherent to the sternum, should be clearly identified in the first or second time-out.

ECMO in TAVR

The use of ECMO or CPB is reported in 3.7–10.6% of TAVR procedures [5, 6]. Patients requiring CPB have a significantly increased risk of morbidity and mortality.

One-year survival following emergent use of CPB is 50% and is 50–86% following elective use of CPB [5, 7]. Studies examining resuscitation after cardiac surgery have demonstrated *venoarterial ECMO* to have better outcomes over other MCS devices, such as temporary ventricular assist devices. ECMO rather than a full CPB machine will also minimize volume loss in an unstable patient. In our experience and others', the most successful use of ECMO or CPB is preemptive, using a preplanned short course to assist *heart failure* patients through the ischemia related to valve deployment. Patients with *pulmonary hypertension* may have little reserve to tolerate rapid ventricular pacing. In right- or left-sided heart failure with anticipated instability, a brief, 10–20- min course of ECMO may facilitate TAVR [8]. Examination of *anesthesia induction* may be very helpful in high-risk patients. Instability in heart failure patients with induction should alert the team to a potential change in approach to either anticipate or prophylactically use ECMO [9]. There are case reports of pre-TAVR ECMO as a salvage for patients in *cardiogenic shock* secondary to AV disease that survived. However, as with all cardiac surgery, shock or multiple end-organ failures portend poor clinical outcomes [10]. A word of warning: instability or arrest secondary to acute severe *aortic insufficiency* is best managed with balloon valvuloplasty (perivalvular) or deployment of a second valve (intra-valvular). In cardiac arrest, ECMO may help perfuse the heart and brain while the AI is treated, but it will also worsen cardiac output and hemodynamics. In the event of *coronary ischemia* with TAVR, temporary support with ECMO can facilitate PCI or CABG. Preparation for ECMO resuscitation in the rare event of procedural complication is critical (Table 11.2). Knowledge of the total vascular anatomy will allow smooth cannulation and avoidance of vascular injury. With alternative access procedures, femoral arterial cannulation for ECMO may not be possible. Depending on clinical stability of the patient, axillary, apical or central access is best.

TABLE 11.2 ECMO in TAVR

1. Large, enlarging or hemodynamically significant pericardial *effusion*

2. Patient arrests and there any effusion

3. Pericardiocentesis drains continual or substantial amount (>200 mL) of *blood*

4. Patient arrests and the echo nonfunction or inconclusive

5. The patient arrests during rapid pacing or outflow occlusion with no vital signs at 3 min of *CPR*

6. Myocardial ischemia requiring emergent revascularization

Steps for Emergent Femoral ECMO Cannulation

1. Obtain arterial and venous femoral *access* if not done. If sternotomy is anticipated, remove fluoroscopy from surgical field and obtain access using anatomic landmarks or ultrasound guidance.

2. Using the *Sorin dilators* and a *0.035″ J wire*, serially dilate for either CPB or ECMO.

3. Cannulate *nondelivery* femoral artery with a 17 or 19 Fr arterial cannula. Use the *venous access* obtained previously for the pacemaker and cannulate with a 23 or 25 Fr venous cannula. We prefer the HLS cannula set by Maquet Cardiovascular (Wayne, NJ), which has multiple side holes throughout to allow increased drainage.

4. As cannulating, have anesthesia give the patient full dose *heparin*, 300 units/kg.

5. Usually TAVR patients are not going to be on CPB for a long time. Partial to full flow (1.5–2.5 X body surface area) is sufficient to sustain a patient through a bleeding, tamponade, or ischemic event. If the patient needs ECMO therapy post-procedure, cannulae can be upsized or added and a 7 Fr, *antegrade lower limb perfusion* cannula should be added.

As many TAVR procedures are moving to conscious sedation and in the catheterization laboratory rather than OR, there may be a delay in or reluctance toward surgical intervention. As the cardiac surgeon on the TAVR, you will lead the surgical resuscitative effort and being prepared is crucial. Your expertise in cardio-

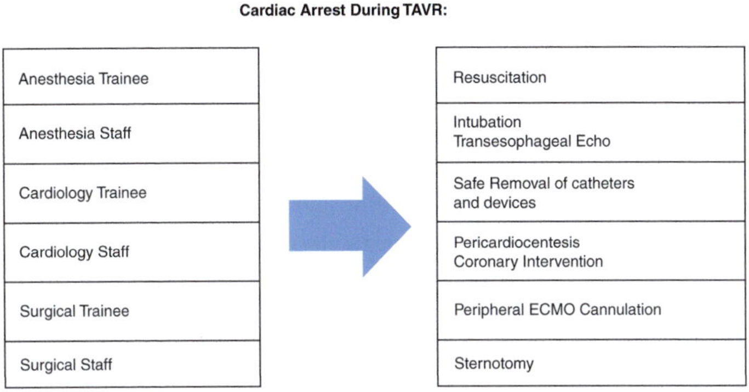

Cardiac Arrest During TAVR:

Anesthesia Trainee	Resuscitation
Anesthesia Staff	Intubation Transesophageal Echo
Cardiology Trainee	Safe Removal of catheters and devices
Cardiology Staff	Pericardiocentesis Coronary Intervention
Surgical Trainee	Peripheral ECMO Cannulation
Surgical Staff	Sternotomy

FIGURE 11.2 Suggested procedural roles in TAVR complicated by cardiac arrest

pulmonary bypass and cardiac trauma will be critical in saving 1–2% of TAVR patients. Including a discussion of possible surgical intervention prior to TAVR will greatly ease decision-making in an emergency [11]. Without clear directives from the patient, cannulate and operate. Below are the role assigned at our institution to best manage emergencies in TAVR (Fig. 11.2).

As the use of conscious sedation increases and more TAVR procedures are done in the cath lab, planning for intra-procedural emergencies will require consideration of intubation and transportation to the operating room. In nonteaching institutions, staff will perform all resuscitative interventions. We stress the recommendation to *peripherally cannulate prior to sternotomy,* not just for reoperative patients or when fewer operators, but in all resuscitative attempts. Especially when access is already obtained, cannulation will provide faster stabilization of hemodynamics. Peripheral cannulation will also decrease the blood pressure and exsanguination through any cardiac injuries found upon sternotomy.

Surgical TAVR Explantation

Several reports describe aortic valve surgery following TAVR. As TAVR use is increasing in intermediate- and low-risk patients, the occasion for explant may increase (Table 11.3).

Table 11.3 Indications for TAVR explant

Prosthetic valve endocarditis
Contained annular rupture
Aortic annulus or root pseudoaneurysm
Valve degeneration
Perivalvular leak with ventricular dilation and dysfunction

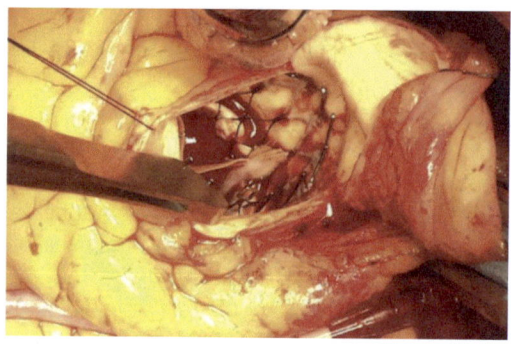

FIGURE 11.3 TAVR explantation [14]

Reports described being able to palpate the stent frame of the TAVR valve within the aorta and an adequate dissection plane to remove the endothelialized stent with a spatula. Others describe threading suture through the paddles of a CoreValve and partially "recapturing" to valve to dissect away from the aorta (Fig. 11.3). While the stent frame may be free of intimal attachments within the sinus of Valsalva, a Bentall aortic root replacement may or may not need to be done. While high risk, these procedures are reported with good outcome between 2 months and 5 years after TAVR [12–14].

References

1. Walther T, Hamm CW, Schuler G, Berkowitsch A, Kötting J, Mangner N, Mudra H, Beckmann A, Cremer J, Welz A, Lange R, Kuck KH, Mohr FW, Möllmann H. GARY executive board. Perioperative results and complications in 15,964 Transcatheter

aortic valve replacements: prospective data from the GARY registry. J Am Coll Cardiol. 2015;65(20):2173–80.

2. Langer NB, Hamid NB, Nazif TM, Khalique OK, Vahl TP, White J, Terre J, Hastings R, Leung D, Hahn RT, Leon M, Kodali S, George I. Injuries to the aorta, aortic annulus, and left ventricle during Transcatheter aortic valve replacement: management and outcomes. Circ Cardiovasc Interv. 2017;10(1):pii: e004735.

3. Pasic M, Unbehaun A, Buz S, Drews T, Hetzer R. Annular rupture during transcatheter aortic valve replacement: classification, pathophysiology, diagnostics, treatment approaches, and prevention. JACC Cardiovasc Interv. 2015;8(1 Pt A):1–9.

4. Barbanti M, Yang TH, Rodès Cabau J, Tamburino C, Wood DA, Jilaihawi H, Blanke P, Makkar RR, Latib A, Colombo A, Tarantini G, Raju R, Binder RK, Nguyen G, Freeman M, Ribeiro HB, Kapadia S, Min J, Feuchtner G, Gurtvich R, Alqoofi F, Pelletier M, Ussia GP, Napodano M, de Brito FS Jr, Kodali S, Norgaard BL, Hansson NC, Pache G, Canovas SJ, Zhang H, Leon MB, Webb JG, Leipsic J. Anatomical and procedural features associated with aortic root rupture during balloon-expandable transcatheter aortic valve replacement. Circulation. 2013;128(3):244–53.

5. Drews T, Pasic M, Buz S, Dreysse S, Klein C, Kukucka M, Mladenow A, Hetzer R, Unbehaun A. Elective use of femoro-femoral cardiopulmonary bypass during transcatheter aortic valve implantation. Eur J Cardiothorac Surg. 2015;47(1):24–30.

6. Singh V, Patel SV, Savani C, Patel NJ, Patel N, Arora S, Panaich SS, Deshmukh A, Cleman M, Mangi A, Forrest JK, Badheka A. Mechanical circulatory support devices and transcatheter aortic valve implantation (from the National Inpatient Sample). Am J Cardiol. 2015;116(10):1574–80.

7. Shreenivas SS, Lilly SM, Szeto WY, Desai N, Anwaruddin S, Bavaria JE, Hudock KM, Thourani VH, Makkar R, Pichard A, Webb J, Dewey T, Kapadia S, Suri RM, Xu K, Leon MB, Herrmann HC. Cardiopulmonary bypass and intra-aortic balloon pump use is associated with higher short and long term mortality after transcatheter aortic valve replacement: a PARTNER trial substudy. Catheter Cardiovasc Interv. 2015;86(2):316–22.

8. Drews T, Pasic M, Buz S, d'Ancona G, Dreysse S, Kukucka M, Mladenow A, Hetzer R, Unbehaun A. Transcatheter aortic valve implantation in very high-risk patients with EuroSCORE of more than 40. Ann Thorac Surg. 2013;95(1):85–93.

9. Makdisi G, Makdisi PB, Wang IW. Use of extracorporeal membranous oxygenator in transcatheter aortic valve replacement. Ann Transl Med. 2016;4(16):306.

10. D'Ancona G, Pasic M, Buz S, Drews T, Dreysse S, Kukucka M, Hetzer R, Unbehaun A. Transapical transcatheter aortic valve replacement in patients with cardiogenic shock. Interact Cardiovasc Thorac Surg. 2012;14(4):426–30.

11. Roselli EE, Idrees J, Mick S, Kapadia S, Tuzcu M, Svensson LG, Lytle BW. Emergency use of cardiopulmonary bypass in complicated transcatheter aortic valve replacement: importance of a heart team approach. J Thorac Cardiovasc Surg. 2014;148(4):1413–6.

12. Hernandez-Vaquero D, Pascual I, Diaz R, Álvarez-Cabo R, Moris C, Silva J. How to perform a late surgical Explantation of a CoreValve aortic Bioprothesis. Ann Thorac Surg. 2017;103(6):e565–6.

13. Bruschi G, Oreglia J, De Marco F, Colombo P, Mondino M, Paino R, Klugmann S, Martinelli L. How to remove the CoreValve aortic bioprosthesis in a case of surgical aortic valve replacement. Ann Thorac Surg. 2012;93(1):329–30.

14. Wang LW, Granger EK, McCourt JA, Pye R, Kaplan JM, Muller DW. Late surgical explantation and aortic valve replacement after transcatheter aortic valve implantation. Ann Thorac Surg. 2015;99(4):1434–6.

Chapter 12
Vascular Complications of TAVR

Iliac and femoral arterial injury is best prevented by through-out studying preoperative imaging. It is important to remember the industry recommended femoral size limitations are for non-calcified arteries. You must know the size of the iliac and femoral vessels in every case to manage vascular complication that arise. Generally, an injury will best be repaired *endovascularly*. This will cause significant hemodynamic compromise, and hemostasis with a balloon dilation catheter will be achieved faster than an open retroperitoneal exposure. Often an iliac injury will be somewhat tamponaded by the retroperitoneum, allowing endovascular repair. (Fig. 12.1) This effect will be lost with opening the retroperitoneal space and could result in arrest from exsanguination prior to control of the injured blood vessel. On the other hand, small, atherosclerotic femoral vessels are best repaired directly with a bovine pericardial patch. Stents in the femoral position are highly susceptible to fracture and stenosis. After achieving hemostasis, a bleeding *femoral* vessel should be *surgically* exposed and repaired. In circumstances of hemodynamic instability and large, non-diseased femoral vessels, endovascular repair maybe prudent [1, 2].

Throughout most of the TAVR procedure, you will have bilateral wire access from the femoral arteries to the thoracic aorta. When confronted with a possible vascular injury, *maintain wire access* across the injured vessel.

© Springer International Publishing AG, part of Springer Nature 2018
A. C. Watkins et al., *Transcatheter Aortic Valve Replacement*,
https://doi.org/10.1007/978-3-319-93396-2_12

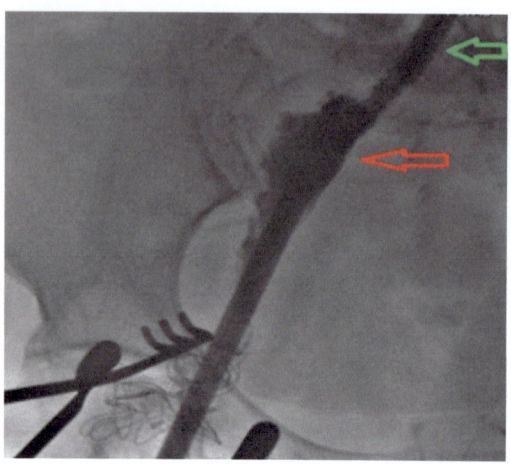

FIGURE 12.1 Iliac artery rupture following TAVR. (Reprinted with permission from Mangla [3])

Whenever an iliac or femoral arterial injury is suspected, the first step is an *iliac angiogram*:

1. Benson wire up the contralateral, femoral artery to the abdominal aorta. Trail an Omni Flush catheter over the Benson.
2. At the aortic bifurcation, pull back the Benson to release the curve in the Omni catheter and point it toward to delivery iliac artery.
3. Shoot a hand-injected angiogram of the compromised access site to determine location of injury.

Following location of vascular injury, the next step is to *achieve hemostasis*:

1. If bleeding or arterial injury occurs during sheath removal or arterial closure: *put the large-bore sheath back in*. This can serve to tamponade the injury and stabilize the patient. This may be done before or after diagnostic angiogram depending on the situation.
2. Either iliac or femoral endovascular hemostasis can be achieve with a *long balloon* inflated across the injury. If you

cannot cover the injury entirely, inflate a balloon proximally and attempt open exposure to achieve hemostasis. Any peripheral arterial balloon dilation catheter will suffice. We use the Mustang® balloon dilation catheter (Boston Scientific, Canton, MA) (Fig. 12.2) for femoral and iliac injuries. Alternatively, an Armada™ angioplasty catheter (Abbott Vascular, Santa Clara, CA) also works well. Depending on location and degree of injury, a Coda® Balloon (Cook Medical, Bloomington, IN) can be inflated in the abdominal aorta to achieve hemostasis.

3. The next step is *vascular repair*. Depending on the injury and your skill set, approach will vary. If the patient stability permits, consultation from a *vascular surgeon* is recommended. For iliac injuries, place a *covered stent* across the injury. Any appropriately sized, covered stent can be used. We use the balloon-expandable Gore® Viabahn® stent (Gore Medical Flagstaff, AZ) (Fig. 12.3). To size appropriately, use a balloon or stent *2 mm larger* than the iliac vessel and *1 mm larger* than the femoral. Again femoral injuries are best repaired with open patch arterioplasty.

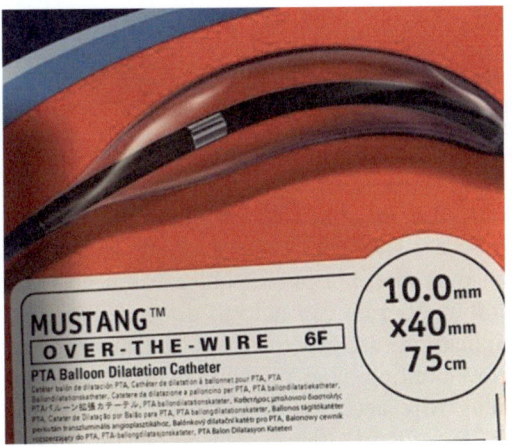

FIGURE 12.2 Mustang® balloon dilation catheter. (Boston Scientific, Canton, MA)

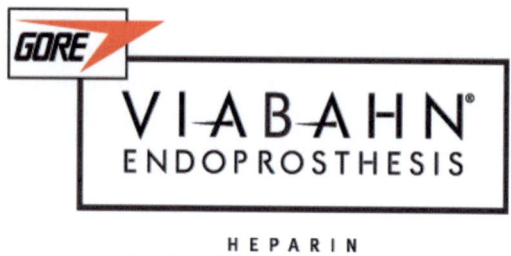

FIGURE 12.3 Balloon-expandable Gore® Viabahn® stent. (Gore Medical Flagstaff, AZ)

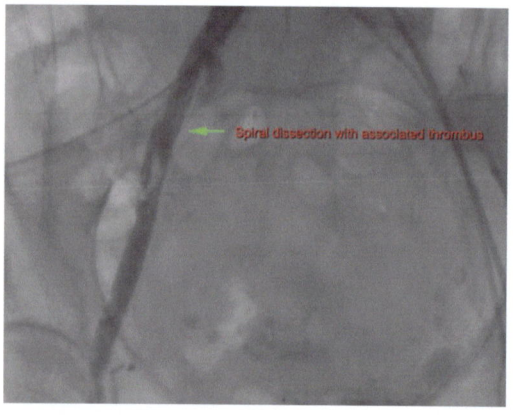

FIGURE 12.4 Iliac artery dissection follow TAVR (Reprinted with permission from Mangla [3])

Arterial *embolus and dissection* also complicate TAVR with any access site (Fig. 12.4). Prompt diagnosis is key to successful outcome. Peripheral pulse exam and completion iliofemoral angiogram can help to diagnose peripheral arterial complications before the patient leaves the operating room. Flow-limiting iliac dissections will require stenting. Maintaining wire access across a dissection will greatly aid in repair. Peripheral emboli causing acute limb ischemia will require either endovascular or open embolectomy. Consultation with vascular surgery is recommended for all ischemic complications following TAVR.

References

1. Thourani VH, Kodali S, Makkar RR, Herrmann HC, Williams M, Babaliaros V, Smalling R, Lim S, Malaisrie SC, Kapadia S, Szeto WY, Greason KL, Kereiakes D, Ailawadi G, Whisenant BK, Devireddy C, Leipsic J, Hahn RT, Pibarot P, Weissman NJ, Jaber WA, Cohen DJ, Suri R, Tuzcu EM, Svensson LG, Webb JG, Moses JW, Mack MJ, Miller DC, Smith CR, Alu MC, Parvataneni R, D'Agostino RB Jr, Leon MB. Transcatheter aortic valve replacement versus surgical valve replacement in intermediate-risk patients: a propensity score analysis. Lancet. 2016;387(10034):2218–25.
2. Leon MB, Smith CR, Mack M, Miller DC, Moses JW, Svensson LG, Tuzcu EM, Webb JG, Fontana GP, Makkar RR, Brown DL, Block PC, Guyton RA, Pichard AD, Bavaria JE, Herrmann HC, Douglas PS, Petersen JL, Akin JJ, Anderson WN, Wang D. Pocock S; PARTNER trial investigators. Transcatheter aortic-valve implantation for aortic stenosis in patients who cannot undergo surgery. N Engl J Med. 2010;363(17):1597–607.
3. Manglaa A, Gupta S. Vascular complications post-transcatheter aortic valve procedures. Indian Heart J. 2016;68(5):724–31.

Chapter 13
Medical Management and Complications Following TAVR

Early ambulation after TAVR benefits the patient at multiple levels, including reducing risks of deep vein thrombosis and pneumonia, reducing muscle loss in the frail elderly, and early decision-making regarding need for outpatient or inpatient rehabilitation services. It also ensures that the patient and family understand that an expectation of TAVR is early discharge, with ambulation a key to success.

Discharge planning should begin prior to the actual day of the procedure, with assessment of possible needs of the patient and family. This includes the ability of the patient to ambulate, need for walkers or other assist devices, and the assessment of the degree of decline and frailty in the individual patient requiring more intense post-TAVR services. This assessment should carry over to the day of the procedure, with the inpatient team discussing discharge plan immediately post-procedure where appropriate. *Pre-dismissal echocardiogram* should be done on post-procedure day 1. This will help identify any early complications and serve as a baseline for future exams.

Medical therapy post-TAVR is poorly defined. Empiric treatment with *aspirin and clopidogrel* follows the original clinical trials, but the evidence for antiplatelet therapy is limited. Concern regarding clinical and subclinical leaflet thrombosis highlights the importance surrounding this issue [1]. Subclinical leaflet thrombosis appears to respond to systemic

© Springer International Publishing AG, part of Springer Nature 2018
A. C. Watkins et al., *Transcatheter Aortic Valve Replacement*,
https://doi.org/10.1007/978-3-319-93396-2_13

anticoagulation. Due to the advanced age and additive comorbidities of most patients undergoing TAVR, the optimal management of patients after TAVR is an ongoing question, with clinical trials such as Galileo, ATLANTIS, POPular-TAVI, and ADAPT-TAVR among others, attempting to answer this question. In patients without concomitant coronary disease or atrial fibrillation or other indication for anticoagulation, DAPT is on-label treatment. In patients with atrial fibrillation and without coronary disease, anticoagulation alone is probably reasonable. In patients with concomitant coronary disease and atrial fibrillation, avoiding triple therapy reduces bleeding, and choosing anticoagulation with a single antiplatelet agent balances risk and benefit. Ultimately, treatment will be individualized.

Additional post-TAVR management will often require standard *heart failure therapy*, particularly in patients with underlying systolic dysfunction and/or volume overload. Symptom relief with a loop diuretic is often required. In patients with normal left ventricular systolic function, significant heart failure may still be present due to abnormalities in relaxation. Co-management with the patient's referring cardiologist and careful monitoring of symptoms at home are key to avoiding rehospitalizations, a major metric of quality and payment.

Fundamental to a successful outcome is vigilant monitoring and treatment for complications as they arise. The most common 30-day nonlethal complications after TAVR in the PARTNER 2A trial, comparing TAVR vs SAVR in intermediate-risk patients, included stroke (3%), major bleeding (requiring transfusions or interventions, 10%), new atrial fibrillation (9%), new pacemaker (9%), and moderate to severe paravalvular regurgitation (4%) [2]. In a subsequent analysis of the current-generation SAPIEN 3 device, these risks had decreased (disabling stroke and moderate paravalvular regurgitation had each decreased to 2%) [3].

Management of rhythm disturbances includes continues EKG telemetry monitoring to monitor changes in conduction or worsening conduction. A *QRS interval > 200 ms* or an increase in QRS interval greater than 40 ms signifies significant conduction delay requiring electrophysiology consultation and likely pacemaker placement. Higher pacemaker requirement rates are reported with the Evolut valves. However, data in SAPIEN 3 valves shows that depth of implantation correlate with pacemaker requirement [3]. Regardless of valve type, an implantation depth more than 5 mm will be a significant risk of conduction defects. Conduction disturbances occurring in the operating room should be treated with a temporary pacing wire from the neck to permit ambulation despite back-up pacemaking capabilities. Patients who are dependent on an external *pacemaker* should either have a permanent pacemaker placed in the operating room or ideally have a screw in lead placed in the operating room that allows for downgrading if conduction normalizes or upgrade to a permanent pacemaker as indicated. A newer option includes the Tempo Pacing lead (BioTrace Medical, San Carlos, CA). This lead provides a temporary pacing wire which actively fixes in the myocardium, allowing for more secure pacing capability at lower cost than an active fixation lead.

Stroke after TAVR can be devastating. Risk of stroke with currently available devices ranges from 1 to 5%. Imaging studies using MRI reveal numerous, small, clinically insignificant perfusion defects in up to 84% of patients following transfemoral TAVR as well as far fewer but larger lesions in patients undergoing SAVR [4]. Risk correlates with patient comorbidity such as history of stroke or TIA, atrial fibrillation, advanced disability, and non-transfemoral device access [5]. Various neuroprotection devices have been trialed during TAVR procedures with mixed results in their ability to prevent stroke [6]. While the highest risk occurs during the procedure, risk extends up to 2 months. It may not present immediately as a focal neurological deficit, particularly in the older patient, but as global depression of consciousness or *cognitive impairment*. A high level of suspicion should be maintained in those patients slow to arouse after TAVR. Immediate evaluation by the stroke service, with possible interventional retrieval of debris after hemorrhagic stroke is excluded, should be considered. The risk of stroke has diminished as the devices have become smaller in size; experience level among operators has increased, allowing for decreased time positioning the valve and perhaps due to less balloon aortic valvuloplasty pre- and post-procedure.

Monitoring for surgical complications in the postoperative period is critical. *Bleeding* after TAVR is multifactorial. The most likely source of bleeding or thrombus includes the insertion site of either the delivery sheath or less likely the positioning catheter. Outside of the major bleeding sources noted in the operating room (discussed above), ongoing cardiac or vascular complication can be responsive to hypertension and therefore present at any time. Any hypotension, with or without tachycardia, requires immediate resuscitation with rapid evaluation for bleeding. Cardiac sources of bleeding (ventricular, annular, or otherwise) are not subtle and mortality rates approach 50%. Rapid pericardiocentesis, median sternotomy, and/or peripheral cardiopulmonary bypass is often required [7]. Vascular injury, less frequent with smaller delivery systems, is still common. Most vascular complications (thrombosis or clots) should be identified in the operating room but can evolve after the procedure. *Neurovascular exams* in the first 24 h following TAVR are critical to diagnose and successfully intervene on vascular complications. Later complications may be caused by dissection flaps that become occlusive resulting in critical limb ischemia or pseudoaneurysms/fistulas. These vascular complications should be managed according to the standard of care. Consultation with vascular surgeons can be very helpful to manage post-TAVR *limb ischemia*. While many can be managed endovascularly, some will require open vascular surgery.

Post-TAVR *atrial fibrillation* is reported to occur in 8–30% of patients. While patient with a history of atrial fibrillation has been shown to have worse outcomes, there are conflicting reports as to the risk of stroke and mortality due to new-onset, post-TAVR atrial fibrillation [8, 9]. New-onset atrial fibrillation does increase risk of post-TAVR pacemaker implantation, although more often due to sick sinus syndrome than AV block [10]. Additionally, there is no consensus for rate versus rhythm control in atrial fibrillation, specifically post-TAVR. Management of post-TAVR atrial fibrillation should follow standard of care [11] with anticoagulation, pharmacologic rate or rhythm control, and/or cardioversion.

Acute kidney injury remains a dreaded complication in elderly, comorbid TAVR patients. Rate of stage 2+ *acute kidney injury* (AKI) after TAVR ranged from 8% to 21%, with 4% requiring post-procedure dialysis. Repeated studies show post-TAVR AKI is associated with a greatly increased 1-year mortality at 55% vs 16% [12, 13]. The most significant predictors of post-TAVR AKI include-procedure creatinine level and post-procedural life-threatening bleeding. Transapical access is shown in many reports to predict post-TAVR AKI, likely due to renal involvement of arterial disease prohibiting transfemoral access. Hypertension, diabetes, peripheral vascular disease, COPD, NYHA class, and ischemic heart disease are shown to also predict post-TAVR AKI [12–15]. Some studies suggest post-procedure AKI rates to be higher with SAVR than TAVR [15]. Opportunities to reduce tubular injury include minimizing IV contrast before and during the procedure and maintaining adequate hydration.

Infectious endocarditis is a rare but morbid complication after TAVR. A large, international registry found incidence to be 1.1%, median time between TAVR and endocarditis diagnosis to be 5 months, and mortality to be 36% [16]. Risks for endocarditis included younger age, diabetes, and aortic regurgitation. All TAVR patients should be treated with prophylactic antibiotics for dental or gastroenterological procedures as done for SAVR patients.

References

1. Chakravarty T, Søndergaard L, Friedman J, De Backer O, Berman D, Kofoed KF, Jilaihawi H, Shiota T, Abramowitz Y, Jørgensen TH, Rami T, Israr S, Fontana G, de Knegt M, Fuchs A,

114   Chapter 13.   Medical Management and Complications

Lyden P, Trento A, Bhatt DL, Leon MB, Makkar RR, RESOLVE;
SAVORY Investigators. Subclinical leaflet thrombosis in surgical
and transcatheter bioprosthetic aortic valves: an observational
study. Lancet. 2017;389(10087):2383–92.

2. Leon MB, Smith CR, Mack MJ, Makkar RR, Svensson LG,
Kodali SK, Thourani VH, Tuzcu EM, Miller DC, Herrmann HC,
Doshi D, Cohen DJ, Pichard AD, Kapadia S, Dewey T, Babaliaros
V, Szeto WY, Williams MR, Kereiakes D, Zajarias A, Greason
KL, Whisenant BK, Hodson RW, Moses JW, Trento A, Brown
DL, Fearon WF, Pibarot P, Hahn RT, Jaber WA, Anderson WN,
Alu MC, Webb JG, PARTNER 2 Investigators. Transcatheter or
surgical aortic-valve replacement in intermediate-risk patients.
N Engl J Med. 2016;374(17):1609–20.

3. Thourani VH, Kodali S, Makkar RR, Herrmann HC, Williams
M, Babaliaros V, Smalling R, Lim S, Malaisrie SC, Kapadia S,
Szeto WY, Greason KL, Kereiakes D, Ailawadi G, Whisenant
BK, Devireddy C, Leipsic J, Hahn RT, Pibarot P, Weissman
NJ, Jaber WA, Cohen DJ, Suri R, Tuzcu EM, Svensson LG,
Webb JG, Moses JW, Mack MJ, Miller DC, Smith CR, Alu MC,
Parvataneni R, D'Agostino RB Jr, Leon MB. Transcatheter
aortic valve replacement versus surgical valve replacement in
intermediate-risk patients: a propensity score analysis. Lancet.
2016;387(10034):2218–25.

4. Kahlert P, Knipp SC, Schlamann M, Thielmann M, Al-Rashid
F, Weber M, Johansson U, Wendt D, Jakob HG, Forsting M,
Sack S, Erbel R, Eggebrecht H. Silent and apparent cerebral
ischemia after percutaneous transfemoral aortic valve implanta-
tion: a diffusion-weighted magnetic resonance imaging study.
Circulation. 2010;121(7):870–8.

5. Miller DC, Blackstone EH, Mack MJ, Svensson LG, Kodali SK,
Kapadia S, Rajeswaran J, Anderson WN, Moses JW, Tuzcu EM,
Webb JG, Leon MB, Smith CR, PARTNER Trial Investigators
and Patients, PARTNER Stroke Substudy Writing Group and
Executive Committee. Transcatheter (TAVR) versus surgical
(AVR) aortic valve replacement: occurrence, hazard, risk factors,
and consequences of neurologic events in the PARTNER trial. J
Thorac Cardiovasc Surg. 2012;143(4):832–843.e13.

6. Van Mieghem NM, Schipper ME, Ladich E, Faqiri E, van der
Boon R, Randjgari A, Schultz C, Moelker A, van Geuns RJ,
Otsuka F, Serruys PW, Virmani R, de Jaegere PP. Histopathology
of embolic debris captured during transcatheter aortic valve
replacement. Circulation. 2013;127(22):2194–201.

7. Pasic M, Unbehaun A, Buz S, Drews T, Hetzer R. Annular rupture during transcatheter aortic valve replacement: classification, pathophysiology, diagnostics, treatment approaches, and prevention. JACC Cardiovasc Interv. 2015;8(1 Pt A):1–9.

8. Yankelson L, Steinvil A, Gershovitz L, Leshem-Rubinow E, Furer A, Viskin S, Keren G, Banai S, Finkelstein A. Atrial fibrillation, stroke, and mortality rates after transcatheter aortic valve implantation. Am J Cardiol. 2014;114(12):1861–6.

9. Amat-Santos IJ, Rodés-Cabau J, Urena M, DeLarochellière R, Doyle D, Bagur R, Villeneuve J, Côté M, Nombela-Franco L, Philippon F, Pibarot P, Dumont E. Incidence, predictive factors, and prognostic value of new-onset atrial fibrillation following transcatheter aortic valve implantation. J Am Coll Cardiol. 2012;59(2):178–88.

10. Biviano AB, Nazif T, Dizon J, Garan H, Abrams M, Fleitman J, Hassan D, Kapadia S, Babaliaros V, Xu K, Rodes-Cabau J, Szeto WY, Fearon WF, Dvir D, Dewey T, Williams M, Kindsvater S, Mack MJ, Webb JG, Miller CD, Smith CR, Leon MB, Kodali S. Atrial fibrillation is associated with increased pacemaker implantation rates in the placement of AoRTic transcatheter valve (PARTNER) trial. J Atr Fibrillation. 2017;10(1):1494.

11. January CT, Wann LS, Alpert JS, Calkins H, Cigarroa JE, Cleveland JC Jr, Conti JB, Ellinor PT, Ezekowitz MD, Field ME, Murray KT, Sacco RL, Stevenson WG, Tchou PJ, Tracy CM, Yancy CW. ACC/AHA task force members. 2014 AHA/ACC/HRS guideline for the management of patients with atrial fibrillation: a report of the American College of Cardiology/American Heart Association task force on practice guidelines and the Heart Rhythm Society. Circulation. 2014;130(23):e199–267.

12. Généreux P, Kodali SK, Green P, Paradis JM, Daneault B, Rene G, Hueter I, Georges I, Kirtane A, Hahn RT, Smith C, Leon MB, Williams MR. Incidence and effect of acute kidney injury after transcatheter aortic valve replacement using the new valve academic research consortium criteria. Am J Cardiol. 2013 Jan 1;111(1):100–5.

13. Koifman E, Segev A, Fefer P, Barbash I, Sabbag A, Medvedovsky D, Spiegelstein D, Hamdan A, Hay I, Raanani E, Goldenberg I, Guetta V. Comparison of acute kidney injury classifications in patients undergoing transcatheter aortic valve implantation: predictors and long-term outcomes. Catheter Cardiovasc Interv. 2016;87(3):523–31.

14. Wang J, Yu W, Zhou Y, Yang Y, Li C, Liu N, Hou X, Wang L. Independent risk factors contributing to acute kidney injury according to updated valve academic research consortium-2 criteria after Transcatheter aortic valve implantation: a meta-analysis and meta-regression of 13 studies. J Cardiothorac Vasc Anesth. 2017;31(3):816–26.

15. Conte JV, Hermiller J Jr, Resar JR, Deeb GM, Gleason TG, Adams DH, Popma JJ, Yakubov SJ, Watson D, Guo J, Zorn GL 3rd, Reardon MJ. Complications after self-expanding trans-catheter or surgical aortic valve replacement. Semin Thorac Cardiovasc Surg. 2017;29(3):321–30.

16. Regueiro A, Linke A, Latib A, Ihlemann N, Urena M, Walther T, Husser O, Herrmann HC, Nombela-Franco L, Cheema AN, Le Breton H, Stortecky, Kapadia S, Bartorelli AL, Sinning JM, Amat-Santos I, Munoz-Garcia A, Lerakis S, Gutiérrez-Ibanes E, Abdel-Wahab M, Tchetche D, Testa L, Eltchaninoff H, Livi U, Castillo JC, Jilaihawi H, Webb JG, Barbanti M, Kodali S, de Brito FS Jr, Ribeiro HB, Miceli A, Fiorina C, Dato GM, Rosato F, Serra V, Masson JB, Wijeysundera HC, Mangione JA, Ferreira MC, Lima VC, Carvalho LA, Abizaid A, Marino MA, Esteves V, Andrea JC, Giannini F, Messika-Zeitoun D, Himbert D, Kim WK, Pellegrini C, Auffret V, Nietlispach F, Pilgrim T, Durand E, Lisko J, Makkar RR, Lemos PA, Leon MB, Puri R, San Roman A, Vahanian A, Søndergaard L, Mangner N, Rodés-Cabau J. Association between transcatheter aortic valve replacement and subsequent infective endocarditis and in-hospital death. JAMA. 2016;316(10):1083–92.

Chapter 14
Conscious Sedation for TAVR

Recently, an assessment of the TVT registry found that from a low starting point, conscious sedation penetration has increased substantially with 20% of cases in 2015 using conscious sedation. Intriguingly, after adjustment for multiple risks, there was a significant *reduction in mortality* in patients undergoing conscious sedation vs general anesthesia. To prevent 1 inhospital death, 110 patients would need to be treated with conscious sedation as opposed to general anesthesia; at 1 month, the NNT was 59 [1]. There were also substantial associations with reductions in length of stay, inotrope requirements, and ICU stay requirements. As it is unlikely to ever be interrogated in a randomized trial, a collaborative approach with cardiac anesthesia to transition from general anesthesia to conscious sedation with increasing comfort level as experience grows should result in increased patient satisfaction with the potential for improved outcomes.

Contraindications to conscious sedation	
Inability to lay flat	High procedural complexity
Difficult airway	Extended TEE use
	Uncertain sizing
Alternative or difficult access	Difficult anatomy/bicuspid AV
Morbid obesity	Study protocol

© Springer International Publishing AG, part of Springer Nature 2018
A. C. Watkins et al., *Transcatheter Aortic Valve Replacement*,
https://doi.org/10.1007/978-3-319-93396-2_14

References

1. Hyman MC, Vemulapalli S, Szeto WY, Stebbins A, Patel PA, Matsouaka RA, Herrmann HC, Anwaruddin S, Kobayashi T, Desai ND, Vallabhajosyula P, McCarthy FH, Li R, Bavaria JE, Giri J. Conscious sedation versus general anesthesia for transcatheter aortic valve replacement: insights from the National Cardiovascular Data Registry Society of thoracic surgeons/ American College of Cardiology Transcatheter Valve Therapy Registry. Circulation. 2017;136(22):2132–40.

Chapter 15
Durability of TAVR

Early TAVR trials were performed in patients who were considered to be in extreme or high risk for cardiac surgery. The comorbid conditions coexistent in these patients were the most common cause of death after valve replacement. The PARTNER investigators interrogated the broad PARTNER database (both randomized and registry) for patients who had survived out to 5 years with over 400 patients treated with TAVR and 49 treated with TAVR [1]. This complex analysis found that surgical valves showed no structural deterioration over time. The SAPIEN valves showed small increases in paravalvular regurgitation. Over a 5-year period, 0.8% of TAVR patients and 0.3% of SAVR patients required re-intervention, of which only 1/5 required re-intervention due to structural deterioration. The Clinical Service Project registry presented data up to 9 years in patients from Italy at EuroPCR 2017 [2]. This CoreValve registry found an annual event rate of 0.2–1.5%, with 20 prosthesis-related events occurring out to 7 years, with no further events after 7 years. The overall mortality at 7 years was 68%, demonstrating the high intrinsic risk of the population. Ongoing trials in the low-risk patients' population, with mandatory 10-year follow-up, should provide the most robust evaluation of valve durability available.

© Springer International Publishing AG, part of Springer Nature 2018
A. C. Watkins et al., *Transcatheter Aortic Valve Replacement*, https://doi.org/10.1007/978-3-319-93396-2_15

References

1. Douglas PS, Leon MB, Mack MJ, Svensson LG, Webb JG, Hahn RT, Pibarot P, Weissman NJ, Miller DC, Kapadia S, Herrmann HC, Kodali SK, Makkar RR, Thourani VH, Lerakis S, Lowry AM, Rajeswaran J, Finn MT, Alu MC, Smith CR, Blackstone EH. Longitudinal hemodynamics of transcatheter and surgical aortic valves in the PARTNER trial. JAMA Cardiol. 2017;2(11):1197–206.
2. https://www.tctmd.com/news/tavr-durability-some-reassurances-corevalve-trials-out-9-years.

Chapter 16
Interesting and Complicated Cases

Ventricular Perforation

A 94-year-old man with severe aortic stenosis and STS risk score of 13% and hospitalized with heart failure was referred for TAVR. He had normal left ventricular ejection fraction, moderate MR, and a mean gradient of 48 mmHg. His CTA was consistent with a SAPIEN THV 26 mm valve. He underwent cutdown of the right groin, with the delivery sheath placed on that side over a double curve Lunderquist. After crossing the valve, an Amplatz Extra Stiff wire was placed in the LV. After balloon valvuloplasty at a rate of 160 bpm, the valve was advanced and deployed. Immediately after deployment, TEE demonstrated no aortic insufficiency, but the patient required inotropic support, followed by CPR, and subsequently peripheral cardiopulmonary bypass. A pericardial effusion was seen, and a pericardial drain was immediately placed. The patient underwent median sternotomy. A bleeding site was found posteriorly in the LV. A LV vent was placed to decompress the ventricle, and pledgeted sutures were placed at the site of the ventricular laceration, along with BioGlue® (CryoLife, Kennesaw, GA). The chest was packed, and the patient was transfused with fresh frozen plasma. The patient was decannulated from the bypass machine. The patient subsequently was found to have injury

© Springer International Publishing AG, part of Springer Nature 2018
A. C. Watkins et al., *Transcatheter Aortic Valve Replacement*,
https://doi.org/10.1007/978-3-319-93396-2_16

of the hepatic vein and portal vein, and due to the advanced extent of injury, succumbed to the complication.

This patient highlights the increased mortality risk in patients who experience significant cardiac complications after TAVR. In a recent paper, the European experience found a conversation rate to emergent cardiac surgery of 1%, which decreased to 0.7% as experience increased [1]. This rate of conversion has appeared to plateau. The *leading cause for conversion was ventricular perforation*, which was the cause for emergent cardiac surgery 28% of the time. The procedural mortality was 35%, inhospital mortality 46%, and the 1-year mortality greater than 60%. This study highlights the importance of constant vigilance for wire placement and positioning and demonstrates that having a less stiff wire (Amplatz Extra Stiff rather than Lunderquist wire) does not necessarily eliminate wire perforation risk.

Coronary Occlusion

A 92-year-old man with an STS risk score of 14% was offered TAVR for relief of breathlessness at rest. A CTA performed preoperatively showed an annulus consistent with a 29 mm CoreValve. The coronary heights were 12.3 mm for the left main coronary artery and 14 mm for the right coronary artery. Percutaneous access was performed on the right common femoral artery via contrast imaging from the contralateral side. The delivery sheath was placed over a double curve Lunderquist wire. The valve was crossed, and the Lunderquist was positioned in the left ventricular apex. The CoreValve 29 mm valve was deployed. The patient immediately became hypotensive after release of the valve. Aortography suggested occlusion of the right coronary artery, as no contrast could be seen in the RCA, and TEE showed a severely hypokinetic inferior wall and RV. CPR was initiated. The valve was snared and pulled back into the ascending aorta. The patient was placed on peripheral bypass. Repeat aortography now demonstrated return of flow into the RCA (Fig. 16.1). The patient

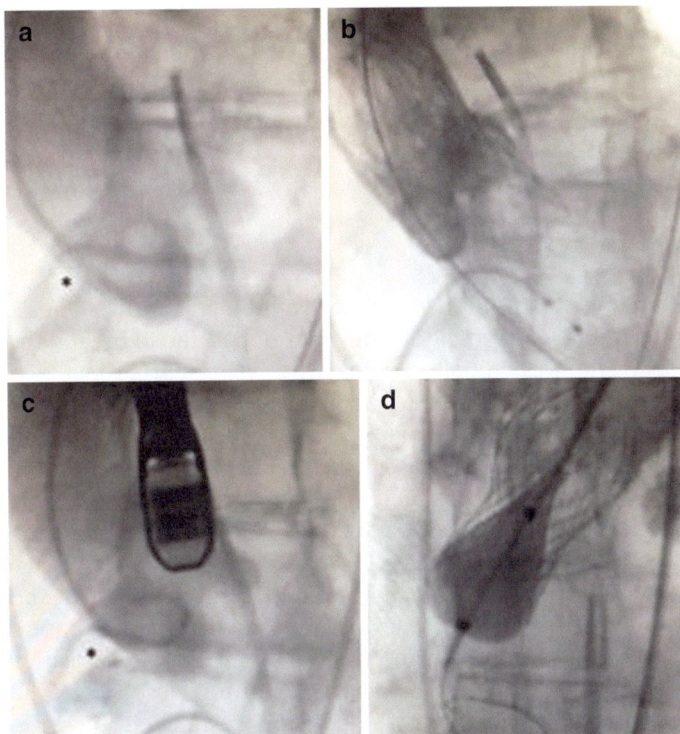

FIGURE 16.1 (**a**) Pre-TAVR aortogram. (**b**) RCA occlusion with TAVR deployment. (**c, d**) CoreValve in ascending aorta. *Patent RCA

stabilized on CPB. The patient was transferred to the unit, extubated, and decannulated. He decided he did not wish to proceed with further intervention and elected to go to home hospice and died several weeks later.

Coronary artery occlusion is another catastrophic complication of TAVR. A systematic review found a procedural mortality of 10% and 30-day mortality of 35% [2]. Coronary heights of less than 10.5 mm were associated with coronary occlusion. The most common putative cause was displacement of the native coronary leaflet obstructive flow of the coronary orifice. Accurate *height measurements and sinus of*

Valsalva measurements are key to preventing these complications. Although *coronary pre-wiring with a guide, wire, and stent* are feasible in patients with low coronary heights, appropriate informed consent should be obtained, and surgical alternatives considered.

Annular Rupture

An 89-year-old nun had severe symptomatic aortic stenosis, preventing her from performing her duties due to breathlessness. She was initially evaluated 3 years earlier but was asymptomatic at the time. She underwent a CTA which demonstrated a cross-sectional area of between 419 and 436 mm squared. There was heavy calcification in the ascending aorta, and it was felt that this precluded her from safely undergoing surgical AVR—her STS risk score was 6.9%. She had a planned TAVR with a SAPIEN 3 26 mm valve after discussion with the heart team. After deployment of the valve and closure of the femoral arteriotomy, she was noted to have a pericardial effusion. A pericardial drain was immediately placed, and 1200 cc of blood was removed. Despite this she maintained her pressure. The decision was made to perform median sternotomy. This demonstrated significant blood around the RV, bruising of the aorta at the aortopulmonary base, with the rupture in the aorta. As the bleeding had stopped, the decision was made to pack the chest. She returned to the OR the next day for closure. She was discharged to rehab and, several months later, back to work in her convent. Follow up imaging demonstrated a small aortopulmonary fistula (Fig. 16.2).

Appropriate sizing of the annulus is key to avoiding annular rupture. The measured size for this patient fell somewhere between a 23 and 26 mm SAPIEN 3 valve. Retrospective review suggests that the 23 mm valve would have resulted in a reduced risk of rupture. Predictors of rupture include oversizing of the balloon expandable valve, heavy calcification of the left ventricular outflow tract, and aggressive post-dilatation of the TAVR valve [3].

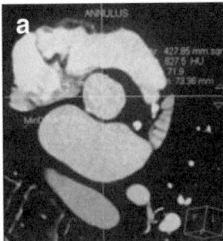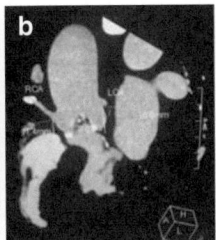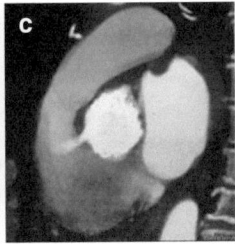

FIGURE 16.2 (**a**) Annular sizing demonstrating annular area of 428 mm² and minimal diameter of 21 mm. (**b**) Preoperative CTA showing LVOT calcium. (**c**) Aortopulmonary fistula resulting from annular rupture during TAVR

Moderate-Severe Paravalvular Leak

An 80-year-old man presented with severe, symptomatic aortic stenosis. He was considered an intermediate-risk surgical patient with an STS risk score of 3.9%. He underwent TAVR with an Evolut 34XL without difficulty with conscious sedation. No predilatation or post-dilatation was performed. Transthoracic echo immediately post-TAVR showed a mean gradient of 18 mmHg. Transthoracic echo the next day showed a peak velocity of 3.6 m/s, a mean gradient of 30 mmHg, and mild paravalvular regurgitation. There appeared to be significant narrowing in the ventricular inflow of the prosthetic valve. The patient was brought back to the OR, this time under general anesthesia. TEE demonstrated an underexpanded valve, and moderate AI both paravalvular and central. TEE also suggested that the valve deployment was significantly displaced toward the aorta. Rereview of deployment angiography post-procedure suggested that the nose cone of the delivery system had dragged the valve several millimeters toward the ascending aorta, out of the annulus. Balloon dilatation with a 26 mm and 28 True Balloon (Bard Medical, Murray Hill, NJ) only mildly improved the inflow narrowing with continued moderate paravalvular leak (Fig. 16.3). A second Evolut 34XL valve was brought 10 mm below the original ventricular margin of the first Evolut

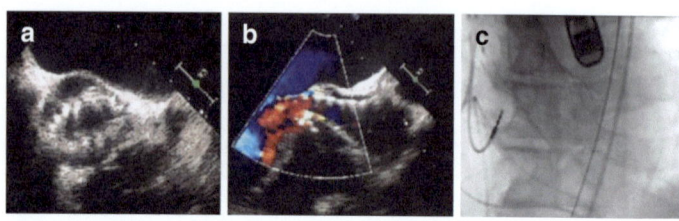

FIGURE 16.3 (**a**) Post-TAVR TTE showing TAVR stent narrowing. (**b**) Stent narrowing and paravalvular leak. C: Moderate paravalvular leak after balloon valvuloplasty

valve. Post deployment with rapid pacing, the valve was 6 mm below the first valve. After deployment of the second valve, the two valves no longer appeared to have a narrowing of the inflow, there was trace paravalvular leak, and the mean gradient was 3 mmHg.

This patient represents the importance of correlations in patients being treated with TAVR using conscious sedation and the minimalist approach. The high gradient immediately after TAVR with a 34XL should have triggered evaluation of why that should be the case. Careful withdrawal of the nose cone of the delivery system, with the delivery wire brought back so that only the soft part of the wire is past the nose cone, may help centralize the delivery system within the recently delivered valve—doing so under fluoroscopy should be standard practice in order to note any drag or friction.

References

1. Eggebrecht H, Vaquerizo B, Moris C, Bossone E, Lämmer J, Czerny M, Zierer A, Schröfel H, Kim WK, Walther T, Scholtz S, Rudolph T, Hengstenberg C, Kempfert J, Spaziano M, Lefevre T, Bleiziffer S, Schofer J, Mehilli J, Seiffert M, Naber C, Biancari F, Eckner D, Cornet C, Lhermusier T, Philippart R, Siljander A, Giuseppe C, Blackman D, Chieffo A, Kahlert P, Czerwinska-Jelonkiewicz K, Szymanski P, Landes U, Kornowski R, D'Onofrio A, Kaulfersch C, Søndergaard L, Mylotte D, Mehta RH, De Backer O, European Registry on Emergent Cardiac Surgery dur-

ing TAVI (EuRECS-TAVI). Incidence and outcomes of emergent cardiac surgery during transfemoral transcatheter aortic valve implantation (TAVI): insights from the European registry on emergent cardiac surgery during TAVI (EuRECS-TAVI). Eur Heart J. 2017:14. https://doi.org/10.1093/eurheartj/ehx713.

2. Akinseye OA, Jha SK, Ibebuogu UN. Clinical outcomes of coronary occlusion following transcatheter aortic valve replacement: a systematic review. Cardiovasc Revasc Med. 2017; pii: S1553-8389(17)30349-4

3. Pasic M, Unbehaun A, Buz S, Drews T, Hetzer R. Annular rupture during Transcatheter aortic valve replacement: classification, pathophysiology, diagnostics, treatment approaches, and prevention. JACC Cardiovasc Interv. 2015;8(1 Pt A):1–9.

Index

A

Acute kidney injury, 113
Acute limb ischemia, 106
AI Index, 89
Amplatz®, 90
Amplatz Extra stiff wires, 63
Amplatz left catheters, 66
Amplatz Super stiff wires, 64, 94
Angiogram, 40
Angio-Seal, 71
Annular rupture, 93, 94, 124, 125
Aortic annulus, intra-procedural
    balloon sizing, 51
Aortic injury, 95, 96
Aortic insufficiency (AI),
    23, 88, 97
Aortic stenosis (AS), 1, 125
Aortic valve disease, 1
Armada™ angioplasty
    catheter, 105
Arterial access, 54
Aspirin, 109
Atrial fibrillation, 112
AV annulus, 36

B

Balloon sizing, 51
Balloon valvuloplasty (BAV),
    20, 46

Balloon-expandable Gore®
    Viabahn® stent, 106
Balloon-expandable
    transcatheter valve, 13
Bicuspid aortic valve, 24, 25,
    40, 41
BioGlue®, 121
Bleeding, 112

C

Cannulate nondelivery, 98
Cardiac arrest, 97, 99
Cardiac surgery, 91, 96, 97
Cardiac-gated CTA, 35
Cardiopulmonary bypass, 91, 98
Cardiothoracic surgery, 1
Carotid, 58
Cath Lab Rules, 68
Catheters, 66–67
Chronic kidney disease
    (CKD), 22
Chronic renal insufficiency, 39
Clinical Service Project
    registry, 119
Clopidogrel, 109
Color-flow Doppler, 89
Confida™ wire, 65, 94
Conscious sedation, 117
CoreValve registry, 15, 119

© Springer International Publishing AG, part of Springer
Nature 2018
A. C. Watkins et al., *Transcatheter Aortic Valve Replacement*,
https://doi.org/10.1007/978-3-319-93396-2

Coronary obstruction, 26
Coronary occlusion, 122, 123

D
Delivery angle, 74
Difficult airway, conscious
        sedation, 117
Dobutamine stress
        echocardiogram, 39
Double-curved Lunderquist, 61

E
ECMO, 96–98
    cardiac arrest, procedural
        role, 99
    emergent femoral ECMO
        cannulation, steps, 98
Edwards system, 13
End-stage renal disease
        (ESRD), 22
Evolut Pro delivery system, 15,
        16, 45, 79
    deployment, 85–88
    Evolut Pro valve, 49, 86
Evolut valve, 125–126

F
Femoral arterial injury, 103
Femoral artery closure devices,
        71, 72
Femoral vessel access, 69
Fluoroscopy, 68, 69
Frailty, 21

G
Glidewire wires, 62, 75

H
Heart failure, 46
    therapy, 110
Hemostasis, 104

Heparin, 68
    reversal, 93

I
Iliac angiogram, 104
Iliac artery dissection, 106
Infectious endocarditis, 113

J
J wire, 63
JenaValve™, 17
Judkins left catheters, 67
Judkins right catheters, 67

L
LOTUS edge™, 17
Low coronary arteries, 45
Low gradient-low flow AS, 39
Lunderquist wires, 64

M
Mammary graft, 58
Micropuncture wire, 62, 70
Moderate-severe paravalvular
        leak, 125, 126
Morbid obesity, conscious
        sedation, 117
Mynx, 71

N
Neuroprotection devices, 111

O
Omni flush catheters, 67
Oversizing, 49

P
Pacemaker, 111, 112
Pacing, 72, 73

Paravalvular regurgitation, 119
Perclose ProGlide™, 57, 71, 72
Percutaneous transfemoral
        access, 53
Pericardiocentesis, 92
Perivalvular leak (PVL), 88–90
Pigtail catheters, 66
Placement of Aortic
        Transcatheter Valves
        (PARTNER), 3, 119
    clinical trial, 4, 5
    design, 4
    low-risk, 7
    outcomes, 7, 8
Portico™, 17
Power injectors, 68
Preoperative imaging, 36, 37
    angiogram, 40
    bicuspid aortic valve, 40, 41
    chronic renal insufficiency, 39
    dobutamine stress
        echocardiogram, 39
    heavy calcium deposition/
        tortuosity, 37, 38
    measurements, 35
        AV annulus, 36
        coronary height, 36
        LVOT and STJ height, 37
        sinuses of Valsalva, 36
    TAVR procedure, 35
    valve-in-valve, 41, 42
Pre-TAVR balloon aortic
        valvuloplasty, 76, 77
Prostar XL, 71

Q
QRS interval, 111

S
Safari wires, 65
SAPIEN 3 Commander delivery
        system, 13, 46, 77, 78
    deployment, 81, 83, 84
    valve, 49, 50

Self-expanding TAVR valve,
        15, 16, 45, 46
Sinuses of Valsalva, 36
Sorin Dilator Kit, 78
Sorin dilators, 98
Sternotomy, 95, 96
Stroke, 111
Structural deterioration, 119
Subclavian artery, 56, 57

T
Transapical access, 53, 54, 56
Transcarotid access, 58
Transcatheter aortic valve
        replacement (TAVR),
        1, 98, 99
    acute kidney injury, 113
    alternative access
        for, 58
    annular rupture, 93, 94
    aortic injury, 95, 96
    atrial fibrillation, 112
    bicuspid aortic valve, 24, 25
    class I recommendations, 19
    class IIa recommendations, 20
    class IIb recommendations, 20
    class III recommendations, 20
    cognitive impairment, 111
    comorbidity, 22
    conscious sedation for, 117
    contraindication, 23, 24
    COPD and, 22
    discharge planning, 109
    early ambulation, 109
    ECMO, 96–98
        cardiac arrest, procedural
            role, 99
        emergent femoral ECMO
            cannulation, steps, 98
    explantation, 99, 100
    infectious endocarditis, 113
    management, 110
    medical therapy, 109
    neurovascular exams, 112
    procedures

Transcatheter aortic
valve replacement
(TAVR) (*cont.*)
aortic valve, crossing,
74–76
Evolut Pro, 79
Evolut Pro deployment,
85–88
femoral artery closure
devices, 71, 72
femoral vessel access,
69–71
pacing, 72, 73
perivalvular leak,
assessment and
management of, 88–90
pigtail placement and
heparinize, 73
pre-TAVR balloon aortic
valvuloplasty, 76, 77
roles of participants, 69
SAPIEN 3 delivery
system, 77, 78
SAPIEN 3 deployment,
81, 83, 84
second time-out checklist,
80
prostheses, durability of, 119
resuscitation plan, 91
stroke, 111
vs. surgical AVR, 20
surgical complications, 112
surgical TAVR explantation,
99, 100

valve-in-valve procedures,
25–28
vascular complications of,
103–106
ventricular injuries,
94, 95
Transcatheter therapy, 25
*Transcatheter Valve Therapy
Registry*, 8
Transcaval aortic access, 58
Transesophageal
echocardiogram, 26
Trans-subclavian sizing, 57
Transvenous pacemaker, 73
*2014 AHA/ACC Guideline for
the Management of
Patients with Valvular
Heart Disease*, 19

V
Valve sizing, 49–51
Valve-in-valve procedures, 25–28,
41, 42
Valvular disease, 1
Vascular repair, 105
Venoarterial ECMO, 97
Venous access, 71
Ventricular injuries, 94, 95
Ventricular perforation, 121, 122

W
Wires, 61–65

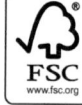